Victor

CHILD BEHAVIOR ANALYSIS AND THERAPY

Donna M. Gelfand
and
Donald P. Hartmann

PGPS-50

CHILD BEHAVIOR ANALYSIS AND THERAPY

by

Donna M. Gelfand
and
Donald P. Hartmann
University of Utah

PERGAMON PRESS INC.

New York · Toronto · Oxford · Sydney · Braunschweig

Pergamon Press Offices:

U. K.	Pergamon Press Ltd., Headington Hill Hall, Oxford OX3 0BW, England
U. S. A.	Pergamon Press Inc., Maxwell House, Fairview Park, Elmsford, New York 10523, U.S.A.
CANADA	Pergamon of Canada, Ltd., 207 Queen's Quay West, Toronto 1, Canada
AUSTRALIA	Pergamon Press (Aust.) Pty. Ltd., 19a Boundary Street, Rushcutters Bay, N.S.W. 2011, Australia
FRANCE	Pergamon Press SARL, 24 rue des Ecoles, 75240 Paris, Cedex 05, France
WEST GERMANY	Pergamon Press GMbH, 3300 Braunschweig, Postfach 2923, Burgplatz 1, West Germany

Library of Congress Cataloging in Publication Data

Gelfand, Donna M.
Child behavior.

(Pergamon general psychology series, no. 50)
Includes bibliographies.
1. Behavior therapy. 2. Child psychiatry.
I. Hartmann, Donald P., joint author. II. Title.
[DNLM: 1. Behavior therapy – In infancy and childhood.
WM420 G316c]
RJ505.B4G44 1975 618.9'28'914 74-14707
ISBN 0-08-018229-1
ISBN 0-08-018228-3 (pbk.)

Printed in the United States of America

Contents

The Authors

Donna M. Gelfand (Ph.D. Stanford University) is Professor of Psychology and coordinator of the Developmental Psychology training program at the University of Utah. Following her work in Clinical Psychology under the supervision of Dr. Albert Bandura at Stanford University, Dr. Gelfand worked in the Community Mental Health Services in San Jose, California and taught at San Jose State College before joining the faculty at the University of Utah. She serves on the editorial boards of the *Journal of Applied Behavior Analysis* and *Child Development*, and has edited a previous book, *Social Learning in Childhood.*

Donald P. Hartmann (Ph.D. Stanford University) is Associate Professor of Psychology and a member of the Clinical Psychology training program at the University of Utah. His doctoral work in Clinical Psychology was done under the supervision of Dr. Albert Bandura. Dr. Hartmann serves on the editorial boards of the *Journal of Applied Behavior Analysis* and *Developmental Psychology.*

Preface

This book is directed toward students conducting behavior modification projects with children, and toward those who may be preparing for future work with children. The book provides a comprehensive description of each step of child behavior analysis from the selection of a child-client and target behavior through writing a final report of the project. Previously, such guides had been available only on a nontechnical level directed toward parents and other laymen with limited knowledge of psychological behavior principles. In contrast, this presentation is designed for the training of advanced undergraduate and graduate students and for practicing professionals.

Our experience in training students in behavior modification techniques has motivated us to write this book. As teachers, we have long felt the need for a single sourcebook that provides students with the range of information needed to pursue a behavior modification program from initiation to completion. Furthermore, we have observed that students are frequently incorrectly presumed to possess many of the valuable but informally taught human relations skills that can spell the difference between the success and the failure of a modification program. The student sometimes unwittingly and needlessly antagonizes his* child-client's parents or teachers by failing to consult with them closely enough and to involve them sufficiently in the treatment effort.

*Throughout this discussion, the therapist and the student will be referred to in the masculine gender. This practice is followed for simplicity of exposition and does not imply that these roles are not equally applicable to women.

This book tells the student which of the child's caretakers he should confer with, at what point in the program he should do so, and what benefits he will gain as a consequence. We also suggest methods of gaining the child's full and willing cooperation in the modification attempt. Thus, the student learns both the steps involved in the formal modification program itself and the informal measures that can be undertaken to insure that the program is well received by the child and by his caretakers. The student is also alerted to the important ethical issues associated with any attempt at altering behavior.

This book can be used to assist the student in:
conducting behavior assessments,
developing data collection methods,
checking the reliability of his data,
collecting data throughout his treatment program,
increasing the rate of desirable behaviors,
decreasing the rate of unwanted behaviors,
demonstrating experimental control of the target behavior,
increasing generalization and durability of treatment effects,
phasing out and concluding behavior modification programs,
graphing and otherwise analyzing his data,
preparing a report describing his program and its results.

Naturally, it would not be feasible for anyone to use all of the methods described in this book in work with any one child. The child-client's circumstances and the nature of his problem will determine the treatment and the assessment methods to be employed. For purposes of completeness, however, we have included the various intervention tactics most commonly used at the present time. Among behavioral therapies, only systematic desensitization, which has grown out of a slightly different tradition, is not described here. Students who wish to learn systematic desensitization procedures should consult Wolpe (1973).

Readers with limited objectives will wish to study only particular chapters or sections of this book. For example, the student training to become an observer-technician will be primarily interested in Chapters 3, 7, and 8, which present information on data collection, observation techniques, and reliability assessment. The person who will work directly with children, but under the direction of others who actually plan the treatment program, will find descriptions of particular behavior modification techniques in Chapters 2, 5, 6, and 9. The evaluation specialist interested in acquiring the techniques necessary to plan and implement a demonstration of treatment efficacy will find the relevant material in Chapters 2, 3, 4, 7, 8, and 10. The more highly specialized, technical discussions in these chapters appear in reduced type. Finally, those who aspire to become thoroughly prepared child behavior analysts and practitioners, and who wish to instruct and supervise others, will want to master all aspects of the complete modification program. For this ambitious undertaking, we recommend coverage of the entire book.

We recognize that many behavior modification programs are planned by professional therapists but are actually carried out by parents, teachers, and other socializing agents in the child's natural environment (see Tharp and Wetzel [1969] for an excellent description of this type of intervention). We believe that extensive first hand experience in working with children should precede advising others in how to do so. Otherwise, the therapist might lack the experience necessary to devise both feasible and effective intervention programs for use by nonprofessionals. Accordingly, this book is directed toward training students in the actual administration of modification programs. However, those who wish to guide others in modification efforts will also find useful procedural information in these pages.

Probe questions and progress checks permit both students and instructor to evaluate the student's grasp of the material presented. A checklist is also provided to remind the student to complete each required step in his modification project.

Our presentation is not intended to supplant in-person supervision by a qualified person trained in behavior analysis techniques, and it should not be used independently by unsupervised persons inexperienced in behavior modification. Close and continuing supervision will benefit and protect both student therapist and client.

Prerequisites

The analytic behavioral approach usually presupposes that the student is familiar with operant behavior principles and that he understands and is able to use basic technical terminology. While we do define these principles and procedures briefly in describing their application, the reader will profit greatly from an extended consideration of behavioral principles – a presentation that is beyond the scope of this book. A sound grasp of these principles will equip the practitioner to analyze the child's behavior more acutely and to plan more effective behavioral interventions than would otherwise be possible. Since he can understand the technical language, he can read the descriptions of related treatment programs presented in the professional literature. From these accounts, the student can obtain suggestions for improving his treatment procedures. And, should his own treatment program prove noteworthy, he can communicate his procedures and results clearly to other behavior analysts. Therefore, to improve the reader's chances of success in treatment applications, we strongly recommend that he have previously studied a textbook such as Ferster and Perrott's *Behavior Principles* (1968), Millenson's *Principles of Behavioral Analysis* (1967), Whaley and Malott's *Elementary Principles of Behavior* (1971), or some comparable volume.

In our own courses we have required that students either complete such a textbook or demonstrate their knowledge of behavior principles in an examination. The student who has accomplished either of these preparatory tasks is then permitted to initiate a child behavior modification project. Those who wish to become more familiar with research on the clinical application of behavior principles should consult the comprehensive reviews by Bandura (1969) and Kanfer and Phillips (1970), and the further readings suggested throughout this volume.

The techniques described here are based on the research of scores of individuals across the country, and would not have been possible without their vigorous and inventive efforts. They are cited throughout the text, and we are indebted to them all. We are grateful to our teachers, particularly to Albert Bandura who played a major role in the determination of our professional interests. The influence of Quinn McNemar is reflected in the methodological and analysis portions of the text. Many colleagues and students read the manuscript and offered helpful critiques. We thank Emily Herbert for her valuable suggestions; for reviewing selected chapters, we thank D. Balfour Jeffrey, Steven Zlutnick, Barbara Hartmann, Paul Whelan, Mary Ann Mahan, and Michael Davis. Pergamon Press General Psychology Editor, Leonard Krasner, and K. Daniel O'Leary and Robert G. Wahler gave thoughtful and thought-provoking reviews, for which we are grateful. Paul Whelan and David Mulder worked with us on the original outline for the book. Grant Number HD 06914 from the National Institute of Child Health and Human Development provided the support for our research, which is described in this book. Our excellent typist and editorial assistant was Barbara Crawford, aided by Terry Anderson, Susan Grant, Denise Kohler JoLynn Skinner, and Wendy Smith. Finally, we wish to thank our families, especially Sid Gelfand and Barbara Hartmann, for their encouragement and patience during this lengthy preparation process. The writing was evenly shared and the order of authorship was decided by the toss of a coin.

D.M.G.
D.P.H.

Behavioral Objectives For Chapter 1

Study of Chapter 1 will equip you to:

1. State the assumptions and reasoning underlying the behavioral approach to treatment and education.

2. Describe applied behavior analysis.

3. Use the project checklist presented in Table 1-1.

4. Locate promising sources of potential child-clients.

5. Use the interview method for study of this book.

CHAPTER 1

Introduction

When modern behavior modification techniques saw their first clinical use over a decade ago, nearly any new application was newsworthy. Numerous impressionistic and uncontrolled case studies of child behavior modification appeared in professional journals. In many instances, behavior observations were made casually, if at all, and therapists' enthusiastic reports of treatment success were often taken at face value (Gelfand and Hartmann, 1968). Therapists presented accounts of the apparently successful application of positive reinforcement contingencies to produce increased rates of desirable behaviors such as speaking intelligibly, completing school assignments, obeying instructions issued by parents or teachers, and so forth. Reports of the dramatic reduction of excess behaviors such as tantrums and assaultive and self-injurious behavior also appeared in the professional literature and received widespread attention in the public press. In only the minority of instances were scientifically acceptable outcome studies performed to establish whether the treatment success was genuine or only illusory.

This uncritical reception was certainly not unique to behavior modification, however. As each new and radically different treatment method has appeared, proponents have at first applied the method informally in practice and have reported glowing accounts of its phenomenal success. Critics have usually pointed out that the therapist's optimism may be responsible for at least some portion of the patient's improvement.

It has been known in medicine that physiologically ineffective treatments can have therapeutic effects. This phenomenon is termed the placebo effect, and it refers to any effect of medical or psychological intervention "which cannot be attributed to the specific action of the drug or treatment given" (Honigfeld, 1964). The placebo effect occurs so predictably in some fraction of patients treated by any method that scientists testing the effects of drugs routinely employ a placebo control group in their studies – that is, without their knowledge, some patients are administered capsules containing an inert powder, or are given harmless saline injections rather than the experimental drug. In the double-blind procedure, the physicians are also held unaware of which patients are given the drug and which are given the placebo so that the doctor's observations will not be biased by his beliefs about the potency of the medication under examination. Only the experimenter has the information about which patients are given the drug and which are given the placebo. Even under these circumstances, some of the patients given the placebo treatment improve. To be considered of therapeutic benefit, the drug's effects must reliably exceed those of the placebo.

Psychologists have concluded that placebo effects may obtain in psychotherapy and educational situations as well as in medicine (Barron and Leary, 1955; Campbell, 1957; Rosenthal and Frank, 1956). Variously termed demand characteristics (Orne, 1962), the Hawthorne effect (Roethlisberger and Dickson, 1939), or self-fulfilling prophecies (Merton, 1968; Ullmann, 1970), this social influence factor seems to account for at least a portion of the success of any new treatment, especially if that treatment is administered by ardent proponents.

When enthusiasm wanes, so does the placebo effect. Thus, eventually each treatment or educational procedure must stand or fall on its actual merits. This is now the case with behavior modification. Fortunately, because of its origins in carefully conducted research in the psychological learning laboratory and the consequent power of many of its laboratory-derived intervention techniques, behavior modification is better able to withstand close scrutiny than were many previous treatment approaches. (For a description of the many and various historical antecedents of behavior modification, see Krasner [1971].) Further, in its most highly developed form, behavior modification incorporates a continuous, objective evaluation of the impact of the treatment program on the client's behavior (Baer, Wolf, and Risley, 1968). Its experimental origins and its continuing tradition of experimental analysis help to reduce the possibility that behavior modification is simply another placebo treatment. One of the most powerful elements of this approach, then, is its adherence to objective assessment and evaluation. Accordingly, we will devote considerable attention to those experimental analysis techniques that have helped give behavior modification its special character.

A number of observational methods and experimental design features have become widely used by behavior modification practitioners. Readers should be aware, however, that the particular procedures used are of less consequence than are the assumptions and philosophy underlying this approach to the study and modification of behavior. It is presumed that much social behavior is controlled by contemporary environmental events that can be identified, measured, and controlled to ameliorate behavioral problems (Skinner 1953). While behaviorists recognize that genetic factors and past learning history are also major determinants of behavior, only the present circumstances are open to manipulation.

It appears that manipulation of the current environment can modify deviant behavior of various origins. In some instances, behavior disturbances thought to stem from organic nervous system dysfunction such as hyperactivity (Patterson, 1965) and seizures (Zlutnick, 1972) have been successfully treated with behavior modification techniques. Even persons with extensive maladaptive past learning histories, such as chronic psychotics (Ayllon and Azrin, 1968), and confused geriatric patients (Swenson 1965), have proved responsive to contingency management procedures. So, while we certainly cannot conclude that amenability to situational controls proves that a particular behavior is learned (Ross, 1974), it is equally incorrect to assume that behaviors of other etiology will be resistant to behavior modification treatment.

The functional analysis of the relationships between a particular behavior and its controlling situational factors is the essence of applied child behavior analysis (Bijou, Peterson, and Ault, 1968). Without such an analysis, it would not be possible to devise consistently effective treatment procedures. Applied behavior analysis permits the user to analyze the environmental determinants of child behavior and to manipulate these factors to improve the child's social and academic skills, thus providing the child with a fuller and more enriching life experience. In contrast to therapeutic methods aimed at producing some diffuse and pervasive personality change, applied behavior analysis (a) pinpoints specific behavioral deficits or excesses, (b) monitors rate changes throughout the treatment program, and (c) evaluates whether or not any correlated changes are attributable to the treatment intervention (Baer et al., 1968). In a typical program, the child behavior analysis practitioner would first carefully assess the child's behavior. He might, for example, evalute a child's speech articulation by assessing the child's accuracy in reproducing sounds necessary for productive speech. Or the clinician might examine the child's performance on some standardized test or against some set of age norms. In many instances, the clinician spends a considerable amount of time observing the child in his normal home or school activities in order to identify the probable sources of the child's behavior. He might, for example, hypothesize that a particular six-year-old girl engages in baby talk because her parents frequently attend to and comment favorably on her speech. Next, the clinician might introduce a program in which the child's appropriate speech earns parental praise but baby talk is systematically ignored. Since he has obtained objective records of the child's rate of baby talk before and during treatment, the therapist can soon determine the effectiveness of his intervention. If the child-client's behavior has improved during treatment, the clinician must then determine whether the treatment is the actual cause of the observed change – he must manipulate the presence and absence of the treatment and observe the behavioral results.

Thus, unlike the less structured therapies, applied behavior analysis provides the clinician with an ongoing, relatively indisputable record of his therapeutic effectiveness. Of course, the same analytic methods described here can be used to assess the effectiveness of nearly any therapeutic method. The only requirements for such an analysis are that a target behavior be defined specifically enough to allow reliable observation and that the observation occur in all phases of the treatment program – before, during, and following treatment. Most frequently the behavior analyst employs a reversal or multiple baseline design in which the treatment is alternately applied and withheld (see Chaper 4 on demonstration of experimental control). If the target behavior's rate varies directly with the presence or absence of the therapeutic application, the clinician can conclude with some confidence that his methods are effective in modifying the behavior of this client (Sidman, 1960; Skinner, 1953). He cannot, however, infer that he can apply the same treatment successfully to a different child who exhibits the same problem behavior. The environmental factors producing and maintaining a particular individual's deviant behavior may be unique. A separate behavior analysis is necessary for each person treated, and frequently is also required for the several problem behaviors of a single individual. Although his previous behavioral analyses provide the clinician with clues regarding the probable functional relationships at work in each new case, he must undertake a separate analysis to make sure that his speculations are correct. To do any less is to serve his client poorly.

How to Use this Manual

We describe the task of the beginning behavior modifier as being equivalent in complexity to a juggler's learning to keep several balls in the air at once. At about the same moment in time, he will have to do all of the following tasks: enlist the cooperation of an agency or family in securing a child-client, become acquainted with the child, select and operationally define a target behavior, read descriptions of treatment programs for that behavior, select an experimental design for demonstration of treatment effects, design a data gathering method, and assess the reliability with which the target behavior is observed. Since these various topics are discussed throughout this book, you are advised to read quickly through the entire book before beginning any part of your modification project. You need an overview of your entire set of procedures before you can reasonably plan your program. Then, as you encounter each portion of the program (for instance, the gathering of baseline data), you can study the relevant material in a more leisurely and concentrated manner.

Having so many tasks to carry out nearly simultaneously can prove confusing. To help you remember the component steps of a behavior modification program and the probable order for their completion, we have prepared a project checklist (see Table 1-1). Each step in this checklist is accompanied by a notation indicating the chapters and sections relevant to

Table 1-1 Checklist for Behavior Modification Project

Place check here when completed		
______	1.	Choose target behavior and perform preliminary cost-benefit analysis (see Chapter 2).
______	2.	Obtain your supervisor's permission to treat this target behavior in this setting.
______	3.	Obtain school administrator's and/or parent's permission to observe child (Chapter 2).
______	4.	Interview caretakers to help determine the nature of the child's problem (Chapter 2).
______	5.	Observe the child's behavior (Chapter 2).
______	6.	State your preliminary functional hypothesis and evaluate your hypothesis with further behavior observations, if necessary (Chapter 2).
______	7.	Define the target behavior (Chapters 2 and 3).
______	8.	Choose a design for demonstration of experimental control (Chapter 4).
______	9.	Make baseline observations and graph them (Chapters 3 and 8).
______	10.	Assess the reliability of your data (Chapter 7).
______	11.	Specify the treatment program to be used; write a script (Chapters 5, 6, and 9).
______	12.	Obtain consent from caretakers, supervisor, and child (if appropriate) to carry out this program (Chapters 2 and 5).
______	13.	Conduct the treatment program, keeping daily records of the child's behavior (Chapter 8).
______	14.	Demonstrate experimental control over the target behavior (Chapter 4).

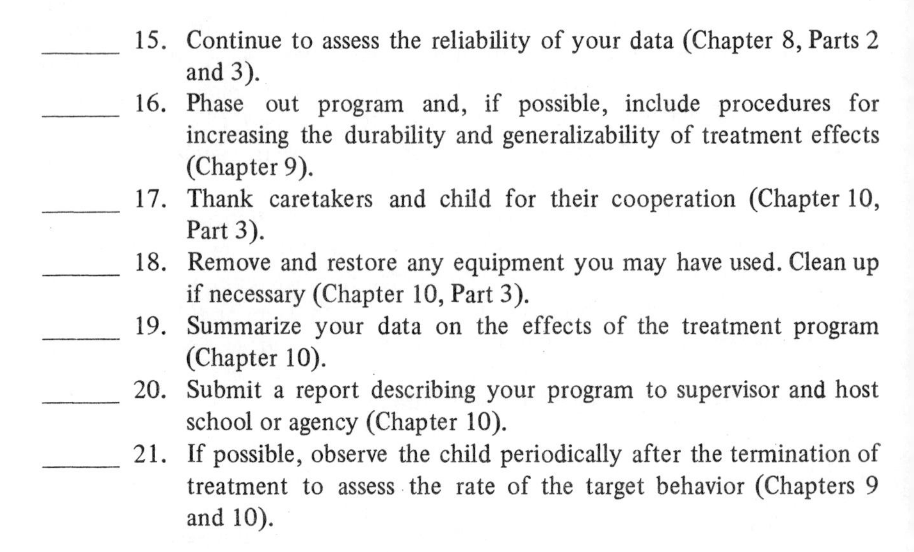

______ 15. Continue to assess the reliability of your data (Chapter 8, Parts 2 and 3).

______ 16. Phase out program and, if possible, include procedures for increasing the durability and generalizability of treatment effects (Chapter 9).

______ 17. Thank caretakers and child for their cooperation (Chapter 10, Part 3).

______ 18. Remove and restore any equipment you may have used. Clean up if necessary (Chapter 10, Part 3).

______ 19. Summarize your data on the effects of the treatment program (Chapter 10).

______ 20. Submit a report describing your program to supervisor and host school or agency (Chapter 10).

______ 21. If possible, observe the child periodically after the termination of treatment to assess the rate of the target behavior (Chapters 9 and 10).

that task. This information should both help you remember to complete each step and allow you to find the pertinent instructions easily. It would be advisable to consult your supervisor before omitting any of the steps listed. When you have completed each portion, place a check mark beside that item. Checking items as they are completed will aid you in conducting your project, and your progress will become a matter of record (and perhaps a source of personal satisfaction as well).

Student Pairs

We advise students to work in pairs in conducting their behavior modification projects. This working arrangement has several advantages over individual effort. In cooperative work the students can provide each other with skill models and with quality control checkers. We have found that a useful blend of strengths occurs when one member of the pair is socially skilled, particularly with children, and the other member has had more extensive experience with operant techniques and scientific methods. The exercises require observer reliability checks at several points. Since each student in a pair can serve as an independent observer, it is not necessary to arrange for some other person (such as an instructor or supervisor) to come to the child's school or home upon occasion to serve as a reliability checker.

Furthermore, since there are two student therapists available to work with the child-client, treatment time can be doubled. Thus, the chances of effecting change in the child's behavior are considerably improved due to the increased treatment-interaction time. Therefore, we recommend that students join together in their treatment programs whenever possible. Whenever more than two students work together, however, the scheduling and coordination problems usually outweigh the benefits; just trying to arrange meetings among the therapists poses formidable obstacles. Therefore, we suggest two therapists as an optimum number.

Should it not be feasible for a student to obtain a partner for the duration of his project, he will have to locate some other person at least to aid in assessing the reliability of his behavioral observations. The reliability checker could be another student, a friend, the child-client's parent or teacher, or – in certain instances – the child himself.

Obtaining Child Subjects

Instructors may want to contact nearby school districts, nursery schools, treatment institutions, or day care centers to explain the nature of the project and to solicit the administrator's permission to allow students to work with the children. Since their specific goal is to modify their child-client's behavior, treatment institutions (such as those caring for developmentally retarded, physically handicapped, or behaviorally deviant children, or juvenile detention centers or state training schools for delinquents) are all likely to agree to participate. Laboratory preschools and day care centers located at colleges or universities are also frequently agreeable to this sort of project since these agencies presumably already have some student training responsibilities in their respective academic institutions. Regular public schools may be justifiably concerned about sponsoring students' attempts to change child behaviors. So, unless the instructor or the student already has a comfortable working relationship with school personnel, it might be better to look elsewhere for student placement.

Students themselves may have some resources in younger brothers and sisters or other relatives, children they themselves babysit frequently, their own children or those of friends. In all cases, parent permission is required before a child can be worked with (see Chapter 2); in addition, whenever feasible, the child himself should be consulted.

The Interview Method

This book is designed for, but not limited to, use in an interview instructional format. The interview method was inspired by the work of F.S. Keller (1966, 1968), and requires that the student satisfactorily demonstrate his knowledge of each portion of the text in a recitation session with an interviewer. The interviewer can be the teacher for the course, a teaching assistant, or another class member who has already mastered the material covered in the interview. This teaching method has the distinct advantage of insuring that the student knows the material and is able to summarize and discuss it.

The customary study and testing methods, which often consist of a student's reading some text material and then answering multiple-choice exam questions, all too often produce students who can neither write nor speak intelligibly about the subject matter. In contrast, the interview method produces students who know what they are talking about. Instructors find that their students' grasp of the material is extremely gratifying.

How to carry out an interview. We have found that the interview procedures devised by Ferster and Perrott (1968) yield impressive results, and it is basically their method that we present here. They offer the following guidelines. The interview should be brief. Ferster and Perrott advise limiting it to no more than ten minutes per chapter part. If the student is thoroughly familiar with the material, he can summarize it readily in a few minutes. If he becomes confused or introduces extraneous material, the interview should be terminated and resumed after he has restudied the relevant sections.

In our own experience, it has proven helpful to provide each student with his own 3 x 5-inch index card bearing his name and listing each chapter and section for which he has successfully completed an interview. After each interview is completed, the interviewer notes the material covered, an act that gives the student some reinforcing feedback and provides a record of his progress. This record allows the instructor to keep track of the rate of progress for his students so that he can adjust the length and frequency of reading assignments if necessary.

Now a word about student apprehension associated with the interviews. Students view most interactions with instructors as evaluative in nature. It is often difficult, especially initially, for them to accept that the function of the interview is instructional, not evaluative. If a student cannot correctly summarize the chapter or answer a particular probe question, he is simply asked to prepare further, then to request another interview. The following examples illustrate correct and incorrect interviewer responses to a student's error in answering.

Correct Interviewer Response: "I don't think that you fully understand the response cost procedure. Why don't you go and read that part again, then come back and tell me about it."

Incorrect Interviewer Response: "No, response cost involves the assessing of some fine or penalty for an incorrect behavior. Like when you pay a fine for speeding or overparking. Do you see?"

Interviewers must take special precautions against appearing distressed or punitive should a student be unable to complete a particular interview, but should matter of factly request that he reread the section. Nor should interviewers give a student credit for a questionable performance in order to spare his feelings. This is no favor to him since he emerges with a false sense of mastery, which is soon dispelled in succeeding interviews or in examinations.

When the student does demonstrate his mastery of the topic under review, however, the interviewer should make an appropriate comment to this effect. He might congratulate the student for his grasp of the material or his understanding of a particular point, or he might describe his progress as good. The student has worked hard and deserves some recognition for it.

Ferster and Perrott instruct interviewers to be businesslike and unobtrusive. An interviewer's function is to insure that the student knows the material, not to lecture or to instruct him. In order to achieve this goal, Ferster and Perrott advise the interviewer to speak only on three occasions: (1) At the beginning of the interview or intermittently throughout to inform the student of that which is expected of him (e.g., "Let's look at the probe questions for this part. Question three asks you what naturalistic reinforcers are and why their use is potentially desirable."); (2) at the close of the student's comments to indicate topics omitted, or to ask that the student elaborate certain points (e.g., "What else can you tell me about setting up a favorable training environment?") or to inform him briefly of points he has misunderstood (e.g., "You didn't get the part about the functional analysis quite right. Let's cover that again next time."); and (3) at the close of the interview to recommend study methods or a particular pace of progress, or to make a general remark.

During a routine recitation session, the interviewer asks the student to summarize a section or to answer selected probe questions. The student should then turn to the relevant passages in his textbook and use the book or his notes in responding to the interviewer's question. The student is not required to memorize the text, but should be able to talk knowledgeably about it in a brief interview. Students should be discouraged from acts of false heroism, such as refusing to refer to the book during the interview. This practice is stressful, and nothing is to be gained by it.

Classroom interview procedures. As was mentioned previously, anyone who is thoroughly familiar with the subject matter of a particular interview can serve as an interviewer. Class members can serve as interviewers for each other. It is often convenient for the instructor (and his assistant, if he has one) to interview several students at or before the beginning of the class period. Those students who satisfactorily complete their own interviews can then proceed to interview the other members of the class. The instructor can sit in on some of the interviews to insure that they are properly conducted and that standards don't vary too extremely among interviewers. The instructor can also conduct additional interviews himself or can informally converse with some of his students. We have found that the interview method lends itself easily to use in a number of different classroom formats, thus providing the instructor many options. For example, interviews can constitute all of the class meeting time or can be limited in duration to allow class discussion or presentations. Moreover, students can be asked to study the reading assignments either during or outside of the scheduled class meeting times. Concerning course grades, the interviews themselves can constitute a portion of the class requirement, and each student who completes the scheduled interviews can receive the same grade. Students who fail to complete all of the interviews could receive correspondingly lower grades. Alternatively, the interviews could be used solely for preparation, and the students could be asked to take written exams on selected probe questions or other questions. Many options are open. The interview method is extremely flexible and can be employed in a wide variety of contexts as dictated by the preferences of the instructor and class members.

Conclusions

This book is not the panacea for the problems facing the novice behavior modifier, but it will provide a systematic framework for his initial attempts. With adequate supervision, the student who carefully follows this manual's instructions should meet with a gratifying degree of success in his child behavior modification programs.

Probe Questions for Chapter 1

1. Why should one probably be skeptical regarding the value of untested treatment innovations?

2. Why might behavior modification be better able to withstand close examination than were many previous treatment approaches?

3. Does the modification of a particular behavior through modification of the environment imply that the behavior was learned? Why?

4. Describe the interview method.

Behavioral Objectives for Part 1, Chapter 2

After studying this section, you should be able to perform the following tasks:

1. Identify and evaluate ethical issues in child behavior therapy.

2. Interview the child's caretakers to obtain *specific* information about the problem behavior – its rate, antecedents, and social consequences – and the nature and fate of previous treatment attempts.

CHAPTER 2

How to Select a Target Behavior

Part 1. Ethical Considerations and Preliminary Information Gathering

CONSIDER ETHICAL ISSUES

It would be incorrect to assume that behavior therapists are the only persons engaged in behavior modification, or that they are the only ones who must be concerned with the ethical questions regarding behavior change. Influence attempts are pervasive in our society. Consider the parent, the teacher, physician, psychologist, advertiser, and even the friend. Each attempts to control the behavior of the child. So each must implicitly or explicitly make a judgment concerning the ethics of his intervention. This is not to say, however, that the pervasiveness of the issue implies that the behavior therapist can escape the question of ethics or treat it casually.

Behavior modification proponents have long been concerned about the ethical issues necessarily involved in *any* attempt to influence the behavior of another person (see Kanfer, 1965; Krasner, 1964; 1971; Rogers and Skinner, 1956). Ethical questions become more pressing and immediate as the means to modify behavior become more potent. Greater power entails greater responsibility. Since many behavior modification techniques have been demonstrated to be highly effective, there has been intense concern over their use. The basic issues concern (a) who shall decide which behaviors are desirable and which should be changed, and (b) which techniques shall be used to bring about change. In many cases, the law provides the answer to the first question. The child is the ward of his parents, and under ordinary circumstances the decisions concerning modification of a child's behavior are made by his parents or by others acting for them – for example, hospital or public school personnel. The matter is not always this simple, however. There are some unwise or even unfit parents and guardians who fail to act in the child's best interests. Caretakers, therefore, cannot and should not carry the entire burden of treatment decision-making.

When the caretakers make a request of a therapist, he is not always justified in complying. As an illustration, let us examine two hypothetical requests for treatment.

Case A. The parents of an eight-year-old boy bring him to a therapist for treatment to control his stealing. Should the therapist agree to treat the boy as requested?

Case B. The parents of another eight-year-old boy bring him to a therapist for treatment because he does not shoplift to help support the family. Should the therapist agree to treat this boy as requested?

Case A seems straightforward. Most people in our society would agree that theft should be prevented. And, since the child's legal guardians – his parents – request treatment on their child's behalf, the therapist is justified in undertaking to modify the child's deviant behavior.

In Case B, the parents are also the child's legal guardians, although their fitness to play that role may be subject to debate. They are presumably requesting the therapist to aid them in the commission of a crime, an unethical and illegal act for a therapist as for any other citizen. The therapist must decline to modify the child's behavior as requested by the parents, and may be further obligated to come to the child's assistance. In these circumstances and in others that are more ambiguous, the therapist cannot respond automatically to parental requests but must independently assess his own ethical and legal responsibility in the matter. The therapist is not simply an agent of the parents, the schools, or the child; he must determine how he can best serve all concerned. Consultation with experienced therapists is often helpful in reaching difficult intervention decisions. Older clinicians will have faced and resolved many such issues in the course of their careers.

A second major question concerns the means to be used to modify behavior. Here, again, the child's caretakers have the right to decide on the acceptability of treatment procedures advised by the therapist. Since they are not themselves expert in the field, caretakers do not ordinarily propose the intervention program. But they can veto any procedure suggested to them. They must be fully informed regarding treatment plans so that they can in fact exercise this right.

Similarly, insofar as possible, the child should be informed of the nature of the treatment, and should give his consent if he is competent to make such a decision. Children who are extremely young, severely retarded, psychotic, or nonverbal are often not equipped to make treatment decisions for themselves, so their parents and other guardians assume that responsibility. Naturally, the caretakers and, if he is competent to do so, the child himself retain the privilege of discontinuing the treatment at any time.

Even presuming that the caretakers and child have agreed to a procedure proposed by the therapist, further ethical questions could arise. This is especially true for treatment based on aversive training methods such as physical or psychological punishment. Most people would agree that extreme measures are justified in extreme cases involving potentially serious injury to the child himself or to others as a result of his actions (Baer, 1970, 1971; Gelfand, 1969, p.372). For example, it is clearly more desirable that a child receive several painful electric shocks in an aversive treatment procedure than that he go blind as a result of persistent head-banging (Tate and Baroff, 1966) or risk falling from a perilous height (Risley, 1968). The discomfort of the treatment is far less serious than the danger of allowing the behavior to continue uncontrolled. But there are many far less obvious examples that require painstaking deliberation on the part of therapist and caretakers. Together they must carefully weigh the risks of continued behavioral deviancy against the treatment-related risks to the child.

Should a child be fined for moving about the classroom when his teacher has instructed him to remain at his desk? Should he be reinforced for quietly following instructions? (See Winett and Winkler [1972] and O'Leary [1972] for a discussion of this latter question.) Should a girl be placed in isolation timeout for refusing to obey a request from her mother? Should her persistent cruelty toward animals be punished or be allowed to continue if nonpunitive control methods prove ineffective? These are not simple questions, and we can offer no simple solutions. No technique can be applied routinely without consideration of the rights and the responsibilities of parents, institutions, the child, and society. The therapist must weigh the respective merits of the arguments for and against intervention and must reach an informed decision.

To help you in this task, we have prepared a list of suggested guidelines (see Table 2-1). Since treatment ethics and the rights of individuals and of society are in a state of transition, this list may not be definitive and may even prove incorrect in some respects. It represents our own preferences and the practices of many of our colleagues. Perhaps the best that any of us can do is to be sure that our efforts to help do comply with state and federal regulations, that the rights of the child, his guardians, and his associates are protected, and that the child receives the most effective treatment available under existing circumstances.

Table 2-1 Ethical Considerations in Child Behavior Modification

To protect the rights and welfare of the child-client and his caretakers, the therapist should be able to answer each of the following questions affirmatively.

1. *Caretaker Permission.* Did you obtain the appropriate care agent's fully informed consent to carry out the proposed modification program? Did the caretakers understand that they could withdraw the child's participation at any time?

2. *School or Treatment Agency Permission.* If the program is to be carried out under the auspices of a school or institution, did the responsible officials give their fully informed consent?

3. *Child Consent.* If appropriate in terms of his age and abilities, did the child-client also give his fully informed consent? Does he understand that he may withdraw at any time?

4. *Consensus.* Is there agreement among those responsible for the child's welfare that the anticipated behavior change is desirable?

5. *Treatment Methods.* Will positive methods be used to modify the target behavior (i.e., those involving shaping, positively reinforcing incompatible behavior, modeling, positive instructions)?

6. *Aversive Procedures.* Are aversive procedures (e.g., criticism, deprivation of privileges, timeout, response cost) to be used only after positive methods were tried and failed? Are aversive procedures accompanied by positive consequation of desired behaviors? Does the potential benefit to the child clearly outweigh any discomfort he might experience? (See Chapter 6 for a more complete discussion of ethical issues in aversive control.)

7. *Protection of Rights.* Are the child's basic rights protected? (These include his legal and constitutionally guaranteed rights as interpreted by judicial decisions; see Wexler, 1973.) Does the child have access to an adequate diet, comfortable and safe surroundings, exercise, education, and recreation?

8. *Right to Effective Treatment.* Is the child receiving the most effective treatment currently available for his particular behavioral problem? (Sidney Gelfand [personal communication] has suggested that this may be one of the client's most important rights and one that is not often adequately considered.)

PRELIMINARY DATA GATHERING

There are many alternative methods for obtaining information concerning a child's behavior. These methods differ in their trustworthiness and in the time and expense they require. Methods in common use include interviews with caretakers and child, psychological testing, and behavior observations. Some form of interview is perhaps the most frequently used assessment technique. The clinician usually asks the child's parents, his teachers, and others who know him well for their impressions of his behavior. These accounts are then checked for accuracy against other sources, such as school or medical records, test results, and behavior recordings made by trained observers. Caretakers' reports and school and clinical records can give helpful preliminary data but are susceptible to halo effects resulting from the informant's general impression of the child; thus, these accounts may prove inaccurate. Psychological tests may lack validity and consequently not yield information concerning the occurrence of the behavior of primary interest.

For the behavior modification practitioner, direct, objective observation is the *sine qua non* of assessment (Bijou and Peterson, 1971; Mischel, 1968; Peterson, 1968). In behavior therapy, a specific behavior is identified as representing some adjustment problem, and that particular behavior is modified directly in the treatment. For this type of intervention, actual observation of the target behavior's rate and the circumstances surrounding its occurrence provides the most useful assessment information (Peterson, 1968, p. 141). Other assessment techniques may add supporting information, but to date none can match direct observation in terms of utility.

While careful and objective observations of the child's actual behavior are perhaps the least likely of all sources to provide false information, observational techniques are hardly free from flaws. Even trained observers can be biased. They can report seeing what they expect to see rather than what the child actually does. Moreover, the observer's presence can distract or upset the child, causing him to behave atypically. In the chapters to follow, we describe methods for counteracting observer bias and the reactive effect on the child's behavior of an observer's presence. There is as yet no really effective method for reducing the high cost of extensive behavior observations. Since they are very time consuming, such observations are fairly expensive. Nevertheless, they are not as costly as invalid assessment techniques regardless of their comparative speed or ease of administration. (See Wiggins [1973, Chapter 8] for a discussion of the problems associated with the various assessment techniques.) On this faintly optimistic note, we shall proceed to the job at hand – selecting and measuring one or more behaviors to serve as the target for intervention.

Interview Caretakers

The adults most closely associated with the child can often provide helpful preliminary information. The quality of the information you receive from them will depend upon their accuracy as observers, of course, as well as on their ability to communicate their observations clearly. In addition, the interviewing procedures you use can affect the type and utility of the data you obtain. The following sections describe methods you can use to increase the probability of obtaining reliable and complete behavioral descriptions from the child's caretakers.

Choose a convenient time. In order to get the most extensive and reliable information from those who know the child, you should choose an interview time that is convenient for them and during which you will not be interrupted. If you wish to speak to a teacher, it is best to do so after school hours rather than when he has charge of the class or is supervising the playground or the lunchroom. If you wish to speak to parents, do not go to their home at dinnertime or any other time when the parents are likely to be busy, if not harassed. It may also be helpful to select a time when both mother and father can meet with you. You can often get more detailed and accurate information from a second informant who can add details an individual might forget and who might be able to detect and modify incorrect information.

Get specific information. The most convenient method of identifying a target behavior for manipulation is to ask caretakers such as parents or teachers to describe any undesirable behaviors they have noticed the child displaying. You should also ask them whether the child in question has any notable behavioral deficits – that is, certain appropriate social or academic behaviors he fails to perform. Once the caretakers have mentioned a particular behavior they would like changed, ask them for more specific and detailed information about that potential target behavior. The more adequate and complete the report you obtain from the caretakers, the easier your selection decision will become.

If the caretakers respond in generalities, such as "He acts mean and sulky all the time," ask them to describe exactly what the child does, how he treats others, how consistently and for how long he acts in this manner, and how others react to him. It is helpful to have them give as many examples as possible, to describe the most recent incident, and to tell you their response. Remember to get the caretakers to talk precisely and in terms of actual, observable behavior. Be pleasant but persistent in your questioning.

The caretakers can give you valuable preliminary data on the potential target behavior's rate, the stimulus situations associated with its occurrence, the social consequences possibly reinforcing it, and whether the problem is increasing or decreasing in severity. If a problem behavior's rate is already decreasing, it may not be worthwhile for you to plan a treatment program to cope with that particular behavior. If it is increasing rapidly in rate or severity, immediate action may be required. Finally, you will want to know what steps others have previously taken to curb the problem behavior and how their attempts have fared. Here again, should your informants offer a generality such as, "We tried punishing him for a while, but it didn't work," ask about the type of discipline they used, how consistently and for what length of time they used it, and with exactly what behavioral result. Child care agents can be surprisingly good informants if they are asked the right questions.

Take notes. Since you will be getting a great deal of information in your interviews with the child's parents and teachers, you will need to take careful notes or to tape record your conversation with them. Otherwise you might forget or become confused about what they actually said.

Questions to ask. Some helpful questions to ask caretakers are presented in Appendix A. Kanfer and Saslow (1965) offer suggestions for further sources of information helpful in conducting a functional analysis of an individual's problem behavior.

If you are fairly certain at this time that you will be conducting your project with this particular child, you will also want to ask his caretakers to suggest stimuli and events likely to serve as reinforcers with him. Consult Part 2 of Chapter 5 and Appendix B for a checklist useful in identifying reinforcing stimuli.

Remember that persons other than the child's parents might also provide you with valuable information concerning a child's problems. You may want to interview his teachers, his brothers or sisters, or other family members, if the time required to do so is not prohibitive. Interviewing others is particularly important if you will want to involve them in the treatment effort. Older, verbally skilled children can also offer helpful views regarding their own behavior, so don't forget the child himself as an information source.

Probe Questions for Part 1, Chapter 2

1. Describe the basic ethical issues associated with child behavior modification.

2. Which persons should be consulted in deciding whether an attempt should be made to alter a particular behavior pattern?

3. What methods could be used to increase the precision and utility of information received from parents and other caretakers?

Behavioral Objectives for Part 2, Chapter 2

After studying this part, you should be able to perform the following tasks:

1. Define a behavioral deficit. Judge the suitability of a particular low-rate behavior as a target for modification.

2. Define behavioral excesses. Judge the suitability of a specified high-rate behavior as a target for modification.

3. Give examples of behavior under inappropriate stimulus control. State the conditions under which such a behavior would be a suitable modification target.

4. Perform a cost-benefit analysis for a specific target behavior.

Part 2. Criteria for Target Behavior and the Cost-Benefit Analysis

ASSESS THE POTENTIAL TARGET BEHAVIOR

Apply Criteria

A number of criteria should be used to judge the suitability of a potential target behavior. Somewhat different rules apply in the case of behavioral excesses, behavioral deficits, and inappropriate stimulus control. Advanced students and professionals experienced in treating children's problem behaviors can employ somewhat less restrictive criteria than those presented here. Their experience should permit them to deal successfully with the more serious behavioral problems that novices are best advised to avoid.

Behavioral deficits. Sometimes a child fails to engage in some behavior pattern generally considered normal and desirable for a child of his age and circumstances. Kanfer and Saslow (1965) describe a behavioral deficit as existing when a class of responses "fails to occur (1) with sufficient frequency, (2) with adequate intensity, (3) in appropriate form, or (4) under socially expected conditions." For example, an eight-year-old child may correctly identify only ten written words (a reading deficit) or he may very seldom pick up and put away his possessions (a social deficit of another type). It is also possible for an entire social group to display zero or low rates of certain prosocial or academically desirable behaviors. In this instance, all members of the group might be considered to exhibit behavioral deficits, (such as failure to attend school regularly), and the aspiring behavior modifier faces a major social engineering problem.

Many students prefer to work with a behavioral deficit problem for their initial modification project because this provides them with the opportunity for learning shaping skills. Furthermore, through association with reinforcing stimuli, the student therapist acquires conditioned reinforcing properties for the child. The accompanying pleasant relationship with the child is itself likely to be highly rewarding, certainly much more so than if the therapist, as a stranger, were to attempt a punishment procedure. In the latter case, he might instead acquire aversive properties for the child, who might try to avoid the therapist whenever possible or cry and show other negative emotional behavior when he approaches. This may prove a highly unpleasant experience no matter how effective the treatment program.

In working with a child who displays a behavioral deficit, your job is to increase the rate of some desirable performance. The following list presents the criteria you should follow in the selection of a behavior to serve as the target for your modification program:

1. You should be able to specify a response that will remedy the child's performance deficit – e.g., that the child should answer questions directed to him by an adult, or that the child should engage in interactive play with other children.

2. The child's performance deficit should not be a monumental one, such as a failure to speak at all under any circumstances (mutism) or a school-aged child's failure ever to walk upright. With such major problems, a short-term behavior modification program will probably fail to help the child to any meaningful degree. A treatment failure may also make the child's caretakers more reluctant to seek similar help in the future, and the untreated behavior might persist or worsen. Treatment of these problems is best left to professionals.

3. The child's performance deficit should be manifested in a setting and time at which you can be present and can observe the child.

4. The child's behavior should not be under the exclusive control of situations or persons you cannot control. For example, if the reason for a child's failure to speak in the classroom is that the teacher or the other children ridicule or demean him, you will probably be unable to get the child to speak if you are unable to modify the teacher's or the other children's behavior. Be sure that you can gain control of the functional environmental variables.

5. Obtain your instructor's agreement to your dealing with this problem behavior in this setting.

6. You should also make sure that you can get the proper space and equipment in the institution or the home setting in which the project will be conducted. A project requiring elaborate equipment, no matter how appealing it may sound, may be impossible to conduct because of inadequate facilities.

7. If you are to work with a child at a school or treatment agency, make sure he has a good attendance record. His frequent absences would frustrate your attempt to work with him, or even make it impossible to do so in the time period you may have available. In any case, it is always advisable to select a second child to serve as a substitute in case the first child you choose as a client becomes ill, transfers to another school, or decides to withdraw his cooperation. If you can identify a second child with the same behavioral problem as the primary child, transferring your program to the second child should pose no particular problem.

If the target behavior you are considering fails to meet *any one* of these criteria, you should select some other, alternative behavior to work with. As noted previously, advanced students and professional persons can employ somewhat less restrictive guidelines should they wish to do so.

Our students have found language instruction to be an especially desirable focus for their intervention projects in that children's language deficits can be readily identified, and marked improvement in receptive or expressive speech can often be achieved in brief time periods. Moreover, few ethical problems arise since speech is generally considered to be a vital social skill and no one objects to efforts to train speech deficient children to communicate. In addition, since schools and agencies have a responsibility to train children in speech, it is often unneccessary to obtain special parental permission for the student therapist to conduct a language training program unless highly unusual procedures are to be employed. Of course, parental permission should not be waived except at the suggestion of the appropriate agency or school official.

Behavioral excesses. Next let us consider the case in which the child exhibits a distinct, readily apparent, maladaptive behavior such as cursing, nail-biting, stealing, lying, or bed-wetting. The class of behaviors is excessive in terms of (a) frequency, (b) intensity, or (c) duration (Kanfer and Saslow, 1965). Use the following criteria to help you decide whether you should select this as the target behavior:

1. The undesired behavior should occur at a high rate, preferably several times an hour. Lower rate behaviors will be difficult for you to observe. If a child has a temper tantrum only three times a week, chances are that you could observe him for several weeks and never have a chance to see the target behavior. If he is in some way reinforced for just one of his tantrums (which is likely to be the case if you are not present to administer consequences), your treatment attempt may fail.

2. The caretakers, and possibly the child himself, should consider the behavior to be at least slightly undesirable – e.g., frequent talking-out-of-turn, frequent out-of-seat behavior in the classroom, eating with fingers rather than utensils.

3. The target behavior should not be extremely deviant or have serious consequences as in the case of fire-setting, self-injurious behavior, or violent physical attacks on others. These should be referred for expert professional intervention. Your course instructor most probably knows your community's treatment agencies and can make appropriate referrals for treatment of serious problem behaviors.

4. The behavior should occur at a time and place in which you can consistently observe it. If you can't observe it, it is unlikely either that you can get a reliable estimate of its rate or that you can successfully deal with it. For example, the child may engage in hair-pulling and self-injurious behavior only after being put to bed each evening. If you cannot arrange to observe the behavior, you may not be able to deal with it effectively.

5. The behavior should not be under the exclusive control of events or

persons you cannot control – e.g., negative child behavior aimed at parents due to frequent, parent-administered beatings in a situation in which you cannot hope to gain any control over the parents' behavior.

6. Obtain your instructor's agreement to your dealing with this particular problem behavior in this setting.

7. Make sure that the child has a good school attendance record and that a second child (preferably with a similar problem) is available to serve as your client in case you must terminate your work with the child you select initially.

If the behavior you are considering for modification fails to meet *any one* of these criteria, inexperienced students should select some other, alternate behavior to work with.

Inappropriate stimulus control. A problem can also occur because a behavior, while not inappropriate in itself nor of inappropriate rate, is under inappropriate stimulus control. A child may display cooperative behavior, but only in the presence of his delinquent gang and not in a school situation. The goal here would be to transfer his cooperative behavior to the school setting. Such a case could involve both increasing a deficit behavior and decreasing unwanted behavior. You might look at it as a problem in accelerating the child's cooperative behavior in response to teacher requests and as a problem in decelerating the child's cooperative behavior in response to his friends' antisocial requests. It is often necessary to work simultaneously on the acceleration and deceleration aspects of the behavior at issue. Whenever this circumstance occurs, review the criteria for both behavioral excesses and behavioral deficits before deciding upon a target performance.

BEGIN A COST-BENEFIT ANALYSIS

If the behavior under your consideration meets the guidelines presented in the preceding section, evaluate the desirability of changing that target behavior. What are the possible consequences of modifying this particular behavior?

Evaluate the Consequences to the Caretakers

Positive consequences or benefits. For example, in the case of a teacher, he might gain more time to devote to instruction rather than to attempts at discipline; he might have increasingly positive interactions with the child.

Negative consequences or costs. Perhaps the program will involve the teacher and will require his time to record occurrences of the behavior or will require him to consequate the behavior in some way. The program may involve disruption of classroom routines or, if the program is conducted in the home, the household routines may be upset, inconveniencing other members of the family. Caretakers may resent their failure in remediating the problem behavior while you, a mere student and outsider, have succeeded.

What imposition on the teacher's or parent's or peers' time and other duties will the program represent? How can you minimize these negative consequences or costs?

Evaluate the Consequences to the Child

Anticipated positive consequences. For example, he may have greater acceptability to caretakers and to peers, and more frequent success in school work, in social relationships with others, or in athletic activities.

Possible negative consequences or costs. For example, there may be embarrassment at being singled out as needing help, time taken away from performance of routine school work or home duties with the absences resulting in performance deficits, possible child resistance to the behavior modification attempt and accompanying exacerbation of the problem.

Evaluate the Consequences to Yourself

Since you will have a considerable investment of your time and energy in a treatment program, you should also consider the consequences for yourself.

Anticipated positive consequences. Perhaps you will find it gratifying to help the child and his caretakers. You may acquire skills and obtain a high course grade as a consequence of completing a well-conducted project.

Costs. How time consuming will this project be? Do you have the necessary time and physical energy? Do you have sufficient funds to purchase the necessary equipment and reinforcers? What scheduling and transportation problems will arise for you and your partner? What would happen if your treatment efforts failed? (See the cost-benefit analysis, Table 2-2, for evaluation of the consequences of intervention.)

The preliminary analysis should be begun now and the final analysis should be completed at the conclusion of the collection of the baseline period observations. Then, if you can honestly and confidently conclude that the benefits clearly outweigh the costs of intervention, proceed to the behavior modification program proper.

Table 2-2 Preliminary Cost-Benefit Analysis

Child Target Behavior: ____________________

Treatment Program Goals: ____________________

Optional: Description of Proposed Treatment Program: ____________________

____

Anticipated Costs:	*How to Minimize Costs* (Aim for two procedures designed to minimize each anticipated cost.)
1. To Caretakers:	1. To Caretakers:
2. To the Child:	2. To the Child:
3. To You, the Behavior Modification Agent:	3. To You:

Anticipated Benefits:	*Decision:* ____________________
1. To Caretakers:	____________________
2. To the Child:	____________________
3. To You:	____________________

Probe Questions for Part 2, Chapter 2

1. Evaluate the suitability of each of the following as a child target behavior for a student to select for modification: (a) an eight-year-old boy's infrequent use of his toothbrush, (b) head-banging and self-scratching mutilation in a nine-year-old, severely retarded girl, (c) occasional (once or twice a month) acts of vandalism such as breaking windows by a 16-year-old boy and his friends, (d) low rate of helping with household chores, such as mowing the lawn, by a ten-year-old boy.

2. In general, would it be better for a student therapist to treat a behavioral deficit or a behavioral excess problem?

3. Describe the potential costs and benefits that must be considered in a projected child behavior modification program.

Behavioral Objectives for Part 3, Chapter 2

Study of this section should enable you to:

1. Make behavior observations without unduly upsetting the teacher, the class, the family, or the child-client.

2. Record your behavior observations on a three-column observation form.

3. Informally assess your accuracy as an observer. Be able to identify sources of observation error.

4. Perform a functional analysis of the determinants of the target behavior.

Part 3. Preliminary Observations and Functional Analysis

MAKE PRELIMINARY OBSERVATIONS

Making preliminary behavior observations accomplishes several objectives. First, it helps to acquaint you with the child and his behavior in the naturalistic environment of his home and school. Second, it gives you practice in making objective, noninterpretive observations of child behavior. These observations, in combination with careful recording of correlated environmental stimulus events, are crucial in performing a functional analysis of the child's behavior. In addition, the functional analysis frequently dictates the details of the modification program. When you know which stimuli are correlated with the occurrence of the target behavior, you can often tell how these stimuli must be programmed in order to change the target behavior's rate of occurrence. Finally, your behavior observations provide some check on the accuracy of the caretaker's report regarding the child's behavior. The caretaker's report alone does not usually suffice, since it is subject to halo effects, failure of memory, conclusions based on unrepresentative or inadequate samples of the child's behavior, and other distortions.

Suggestions for Observers

Some rules of conduct apply whenever you make behavioral observations of children. The following suggestions are based on Broden's (undated) recommendations and on our own experience.

1. Obtain the caretaker's permission to observe the child in his normal social environment or wherever the treatment project will take place. If this is to occur in a school setting, the school principal's and the teacher's permission will be required to allow you to observe the child in the classroom or on the playground. In certain agencies you may also need the parents' permission to observe a specific child. Check with the school personnel to find out whether this will be necessary.

2. *For observations in the classroom,* the teacher may wish to introduce you to the class so that they will know who you are and something about why you are there. The teacher may want to tell them, "This is (your name). He is a student at (your school) and he is interested in learning how to work with children and in how we do things at our school. So he will be visiting with us and might work with some of you." It is advisable to discuss with the teacher beforehand what he intends telling the class about your project, and to attempt to insure that he will not terrify Johnny by announcing in class that you are there to observe *him*. The announcement should be acceptable to

both of you.

3. Insofar as possible, your entrance into or departure from an observation setting should coincide with a normal break in the daily routine, such as snack time, a locker use period, a lunch break, or the beginning or close of a class period.

4. As an observer, you want to blend into the background as much as possible, so be inconspicuous in your personal appearance and your behavior – for example, don't chew gum or eat candy. Try not to dress or act in a way that will draw the children's attention.

5. Do not strike up conversations with the children. You want them to behave as normally as possible, just as though you were not there. If they talk to you, answer their specific questions as briefly as possible, then turn away and busy yourself with something else. Some observers simply ignore children's approaches and continue writing until the children give up and leave them alone.

6. Try not to disrupt the classroom routine. Sit at the back of the room in an inconspicuous place from which you can see but cannot easily be seen so that you will not interfere with the children's concentration on their work. A chair placed at the side or back of the classroom or in a living room or dining room in a constant location maintained from day to day will serve as a good observation location. If you also have placed other chairs or stools at various vantage points in the behavior setting, you can walk unobtrusively from one to another to keep the child in view.

7. To prevent the target child from becoming too self-conscious, you should disguise your keen interest in him by varying the apparent object of your glances. This is most desirable early in the observation process when both you and the child are becoming accustomed to the procedure.

8. Do not begin making systematic behavior observations until the children have become accustomed to your presence. Wait until they're behaving in their usual fashion. This may require several hours or even a day or more. You can, however, practice recording observations during the acquaintance period, and can refine your behavioral definitions and select the optimal time of day to make your observations throughout your project.

9. Take your observations at the same time each day. This regularity creates less classroom or home disturbance and guarantees that changes observed in the child's behavior are not due simply to variations in the time of day at which the observation took place.

10. Thank the teacher for letting you visit, if you can do so inconspicuously, before you leave the school each time you observe. And inform him about the probable time of your next visit. Inquire if that time is acceptable to him. Your project is an imposition on him. Show him that you realize this

and are grateful for his help. Remember, you need him, he does not need you; nor, at this stage of your project, does he probably feel that you can be of significant benefit to him or to the students. At this point, he is probably somewhat skeptical, but willing to cooperate if your project sounds reasonable.

11. *For observations in the home,* make sure that the parents do not introduce you as some sort of policeman who has come to make Johnny behave. In this situation, also, it might be advisable to ask them to present you as a student who is interested in learning how to work with children and families. The other rules for making observations obtain here as well, such as those concerning remaining as unobtrusive as possible and allowing a habituation time before commencing the actual observations.

The Observation Record Format

Your next task will be to make your observations in a manner that will help you identify the situational determinants of the child's behavior. There are a number of antecedent and consequent events that can affect behavior. These include setting events (Bijou and Baer, 1961; Kantor, 1958), stimulus events (potential S^D's) associated with the operant behavior, and consequences that might act as reinforcers or punishing stimuli. For example, to understand why a certain child predictably has temper tantrums between 5:00 and 7:00 p.m. each day, it would be helpful to know that during this time period his dinnertime is approaching and he is relatively food-deprived and fatigued (setting events), that his mother's preoccupation with preparing dinner and his father's attention to the television news report deprive him of their attention (also a setting event). Additionally, his siblings may respond to him in a surly fashion since they are also food-deprived, attention-deprived, and fatigued, thus providing models for quarrelsome behavior (S^D's) and punishing social consequences for the child's interaction attemps. In such circumstances, the child in question may coerce attention, food, and enforced rest from his family by engaging in ill-tempered outbursts.

Remediation procedures might concentrate on setting events; for example, the children could be given a mid-afternoon snack and a nap to alleviate their food- and rest-deprivation, or the family's dinnertime could be changed to an earlier hour to accomplish the same result. Alternatively, the treatment intervention could concentrate on the parents' behavior so that they no longer place their children on extinction schedules prior to dinner. This would involve manipulation of (a) setting events – namely, the attention deprivation, (b) possible S^D's the parents emit – signaling the potentiality of reinforcement only if the child misbehaves, and (c) consequent social events such that the parents reinforce their children's cooperative behavior and either ignore or punish quarrelsome behavior with fines (response cost) or isolation (timeout) procedures. All of these intervention procedures will be discussed at length in succeeding portions of this book.

Setting events. Since setting events will remain essentially unchanged throughout a single observation session, you should preface the behavioral record with your information and speculations regarding relevant setting events. For example, you should investigate and report the child's current condition of deprivation for the particular reinforcer you intend using, and you should know his current general state of health and alertness and the instructions he has been given concerning you and your project. Other setting events could consist of the child's having experienced some unsettling interpersonal experience, such as moving to a new neighborhood, a death in the family, or an auto accident.

Discriminative stimuli. You should note carefully the stimulus events associated with each of the child's responses. For example, in interpreting the child's behavior of walking toward the teacher's desk, it is important to know that the teacher's comment, "Children, look what I have here," preceded the child's action. The teacher's comment, a stimulus event, may well be serving as a discriminative stimulus.

Child's behavior. Additionally, you will require a careful description of the child's behavior. Does he look at the teacher, does he smile or make a funny face, does he dawdle or walk briskly or run over to the teacher's desk? All these aspects of his behavior should be noted.

Consequent social events. What happens immediately after the child's response? What are the social consequences of his action? Does the teacher address a particular comment to the child, give him play materials, or turn away? Again, you must record precisely what happens following the child's response.

This "three-term contingency" (Bijou, Peterson, Harris, Allen, and Johnston, 1969; Skinner, 1953), which includes antecedent stimulus and setting events, the child's responses, and the consequent social events, provides the information necessary to a functional analysis of the child's behavior.

Table 2-3 presents an example of a three-column observation record that includes antecedent and consequent social events as well as the responses emitted by the child who is the primary object of observation. A sample functional analysis of the determinants of the child's behavior is also included.

Rules for recording. General rules for you to follow in recording your own observations in a three-column table are as follows:

1. Describe only the behavior or stimulus events that you can actually observe. Do not interpret or evaluate the behavior.

Incorrect: Tommy walked disconsolately away from the swings.
Correct: Tommy walked slowly, with his head down, away from the swings.
Incorrect: Susan was delighted to hold the cat.
Correct: Susan smiled as she held the cat.
Incorrect: Mark was angry at Bill.
Correct: Mark frowned at Bill.

2. Record nonverbal as well as verbal behavior, for example, if the child is watching another child for two minutes, then approaches the other child and says "Hi," record the watching and the walking as well as the greeting directed toward the other child. Remember that social events can be nonverbal as well as verbal.

3. Note the exact time each time you observe the child initiating a new behavior or someone initiating an interaction with him. Having a record of the time of occurrence of each behavior makes it easier to keep the sequence of the action clear. Knowing the exact sequence is important in determining the situational controls over the child's behavior.

4. Use abbreviations or shorthand notations that will allow you to record all of the action as it occurs. Use any system that seems easy and natural for you and that you can decipher easily at some later time.

Note that since most behavior is chained the consequent stimulus event for child behavior 1 will also frequently be the antecedent event for child behavior 2, the consequent for child behavior 2 will be the antecedent for child behavior 3, and so on. When this circumstance occurs, you can save writing time and avoid needless duplication by placing a check mark (√) in the antecedent event column to indicate that this antecedent is identical to the immediately preceding consequent event:

Antecedent	**Response**	**Consequent**
1. John says, "Mary come here."	2. Mary runs over to John.	3. John hugs Mary.
3. John hugs Mary.	4. Mary says, "Want to play catch?"	5. John nods.

The above example can be represented this way:

1. J: "M come here."	2. M runs over to J.	3. J hugs M.
3. √	4. M: "Want to play catch?"	5. J nods.

Table 2-3 Sample Three-Column Behavior Observation Format

Setting: A cooperative nursery school in which the children's mothers participate on a regularly scheduled basis. There are 14 children between the ages of 3-1/2 and 4 years. Jack is a cute, chubby four-year-old boy whose mother is assisting the nursery school teacher this afternoon. A group of three children are making objects out of Play Dough while seated at a small table. Jack is standing by the table and also working with the Play Dough.

Time	Antecedent Event	Response	Consequent Social Event
1:30 PM		1. J says, "I need a knife."	2. Children ignore him.
	2. Children ignore him.	2. J cries, screams, "That's mine" to girl using knife.	3. Girl ignores him. Teacher: "Sit here."
	3. √	4. J: "No. Knife."	5. Teacher (T): "That's not the decision you made, remember?"
	5. √	6. J throws dough back into the bucket. He begins to cry again.	7. J's mother and T ignore him.
1:35	7. √	8. J leaves room; returns two minutes later crying as loudly as before.	9. T takes J to an adjoining room, and tells him: "You can sit here until you can stop crying."
	9. √	10. J sits on chair, gradually stops crying, then gets up and returns to other room.	

Time	Antecedent Event	Response	Consequent Social Event
1:40	11. J's mother is operating a tape recorder. The children are recording statements of their favorite foods. Mother (M) asks each individually what his favorite food is. M: "J, what is your favorite food?"	12. "Marshmallows."	13. M: "O.K., now let's hear what Cathy's favorite is." (Continues until all have had a turn.) "Shall we listen to our tape now?"
	13. √	14. J shouts "Yes" with other children.	15. M replays tape.

1:45	15. √	16. "That sounded like me, Mom, roll it back." J begins to thrash his arms and cry.	17. M reverses tape to play J's voice again.
	17. √	18. J stops crying. Then says, "What is your ickiest food?"	19. Group ignores him.
	19. √	20. J listens to tape, whines occasionally. Suddenly J begins jumping and crying, screams, "Turn it all back again."	21. M reverses tape and plays it back again.
1:52			
	22. After conclusion of tape, M asks the children where they want to go on summer vacations.	23. J starts crying again	24. T: "Your mother is talking."
1:54	24. √	25. J cries louder	26. M and T ignore him.

Functional Hypothesis: This child's mother and, to a lesser extent, his teacher are intermittently reinforcing his crying and protesting by complying with his demands and attending to him when he misbehaves (events 19-25). More consistent use of the timeout procedure of placing him in a chair in an adjoining room (event 9) combined with adult attention and praise for socially appropriate behavior would probably effectively reduce his frequent complaints and demands. The treatment presently employed by the mother and teacher will probably eventually increase Jack's cooperative behavior, but only after considerable disruption of group activities, annoyance to the other children, and wear and tear on all involved. It appears that all participants would profit from the introduction of the suggested revised child management procedures.

Note: Helen Fishler recorded these observations as part of a child psychology class project.

Assess Observer Accuracy

Perhaps you have failed to observe one or more significant interactions. Check the accuracy of your observations by having a second person independently record the child's behavior during the same 10- to 15-minute period you do. First synchronize your watches, then make sure that both of you can see and hear the child equally well. Make your observations independently, then get together and compare your records. If they do not match well, try to determine the reason. Could both of you see the child well? Could both of you hear him? Did both of you record his nonverbal as well as his verbal behavior? Did you record only behavior you actually witnessed? Did one of you use some form of shorthand or abbreviations that allowed you to make a more complete record? The use of a second observer alerts you to the possibility of error in your observations through checking your alertness and objectivity.

Perform a Preliminary Functional Analysis of the Determinants of the Target Behavior.

Using observations alone, there is no very precise nor foolproof method for determining the stimulus conditions controlling the target behavior. The most you can get from your behavior observations is some indication of covariation of particular stimuli and the occurrence of the target behavior. For example, an antecedent stimulus of taunting by playmates may be reliably followed by high-rate crying in a kindergarten child. Your functional hypothesis in this case would then be that the taunting has produced the crying. Or the child's crying might reliably be followed by teacher attention in the form of sympathetic remarks such as, "Now we have made Johnny feel bad." Here you might hypothesize a functional relationship between Johnny's crying and the teacher's reinforcement of crying. When you rely on observational data alone, you can never be completely sure what functional relationships are operating. You cast your best guesses in the form of a hypothesis, and this hypothesis helps to determine your treatment plan.

To perform your functional analysis using your three-column behavior records, encircle each row describing the target behavior and its antecedents and consequents. Are the antecedents and/or the consequents the same in more than one instance? If so, state a functional hypothesis about the probable environmental maintainers of the problem behavior – e.g., is each instance of a child's talking-out-of-turn preceded by the teacher's praising another child? Is each talking-out-of-turn instance followed by a reply from the teacher or laughter from the other children? In the latter example, you might hypothesize that peer attention is acting as a reinforcer and is maintaining the child's talking-out-of-turn.

Perform Additional Behavior Observations to Evaluate the Validity of Your Hypothesis

In some cases there is little doubt about the probable factors maintaining the problem behaviors, so this additional step is unnecessary. However, when you have considerable hesitation about the correctness of your hypothesis, you might save yourself wasted time and effort by getting additional information at this point. It is possible that more than one type of antecedent or consequent is acting to maintain this target behavior. Does your hypothesis hold up in the light of your further observations? Does your instructor agree with your analysis? If possible, ask the child or his caretakers what they believe to be the source of the child's target behavior. They may be able to provide you with valuable additional clues.

Now you must decide whether your original hypothesis is adequate or whether it must be revised, and (in the latter case) how it must be revised.

At this point you are ready to pinpoint the target behavior and its environmental controls. Your next steps will be to define the target behavior precisely, to gather data on its baseline rate of occurrence, and to plan a treatment intervention.

Probe Questions for Part 3, Chapter 2

1. What precautions must be taken to minimize an observer's intrusion into a naturalistic behavior setting of a home or school?

2. Define setting events, discriminative stimuli, and consequent social events. What role does each play in a functional analysis of a child's behavior?

3. Transcribe the following narrative record into a three-column format, numbering each event to indicate the proper sequence. "Jay (J), a five-year-old boy is in a kindergarten classroom with five other children and his teacher (T). The room is furnished with a piano, a rocking horse, three chairs, a portable record player, and a table that holds various toys. T is instructing the children in various dance movements. T tells the class, "No one is to get on the horse." J climbs onto the horse. T: "Please get off, J." J gets off the rocking horse and T says: "Thank you, J." Next J climbs onto a chair and stands up on the seat. T: "Please get off that chair, J. Children, everyone stay off of the chairs and table now." J remains on the chair. T: "J, get off the chair *now.*" J makes a face and says, "My shoe hurts." T: "Get off the chair, J." J: "I have to take my shoes off first." He takes his shoes off slowly and then gets down from the chair. T: "Get in line." J ignores her, plays with some lint on the floor, and pushes a toy car back and forth beside him. T walks over to J, takes hold of his arm, and pulls him into line with the other children who are doing a march step.

4. Perform a functional analysis of J's behavior described in the preceding passage. Which events could be altered to improve J's behavior?

Behavioral Objectives for Part 1, Chapter 3

After study of Part 1 of this chapter, you should be able to:

1. Describe the primary advantages and disadvantages of systematic data collection.

2. Distinguish between direct and indirect measures of a target behavior, and between topographic and functional response definitions.

3. Devise a target response definition that is meaningful, behavioral, and produces reliable data.

CHAPTER 3

Developing a Procedure for Collecting Data

Part 1. Response Definitions

INTRODUCTION

This chapter and Chapters 8 and 9 are concerned with developing, implementing, and evaluating a procedure for collecting data. This emphasis on data collection follows from the belief we share with others (Franks and Brady, 1970; Johnson and Bolstad, 1973) that an empirical orientation is one of behavior modification's most important and perhaps most enduring contributions to the helping sciences. Because of a popular disinclination to collect and scrutinize clinical data, today's principles and procedures too often become tomorrow's artifacts and clinical curiosities. It is to be hoped that a firm data base will lessen this faddism.

An argument commonly raised against data-oriented approaches to treatment is that they are unnecessary: "If you have changed behavior, parents or other caretakers will inform you of the change." Unfortunately, reports from parents and teachers are notoriously unreliable. Sometimes caretakers are honestly mistaken (e.g., Harris, Wolf, and Baer, 1964); at other times their glowing reports are more a reflection of their consideration for the feelings of the therapist than of their sensitivity to behavior change (Hathaway, 1948). Social convention requires some expression of gratitude to a person who has attempted to help. Thus, the thanks, and perhaps reassurances, of caretakers may lead therapists to overestimate their own effectiveness. Consequently, attempts to demonstrate change or causal relationships are unlikely to succeed unless substantial attention is given to systematic and objective data collection.

Advantages of Data Collection

In addition to the advantages described above, other benefits accrue during the process of obtaining good data. While taking baseline observations on the target behavior, you will become more familiar with the child's repertoire of behavior in a naturalistic situation; you will have a check on the accuracy of significant caretakers' verbal reports; you may discover important controlling variables for the target behavior that were previously overlooked; and you will receive practice in developing definitions and rating scales.

Regular data collection during the treatment phase of your program is perhaps even more beneficial. This continuous record should allow detection of ineffective treatment procedures at a time when a change in tactics is still possible. (This does not mean, however, that methods should be abandoned before they have truly had a chance to affect change!) Daily, or even momentary, fluctuations in the rate of the target behavior can alert you to changes in the effectiveness of your reinforcers, to misplaced or omitted sequences in your programming of materials, and even to mistakes in your interpersonal interactions with the child. In addition, a prominently displayed record of your daily progress with the child can also function as a powerful reinforcer for you and for the child, as well as for the child's caretakers.

Disadvantages of Data Collection

The data-oriented approach to behavior change that we are suggesting also may prove disappointing: The data may indicate that your treatment techniques are unsuccessful or that any improvement that occurred was not due to your intervention. When reliable data are at hand, it is more difficult to delude yourself and to take credit for producing change when no credit is due. Perhaps this explains the penchant traditional behavior change agents had for not gathering data or for gathering data that were sufficiently ambiguous to allow for face-saving interpretations. Furthermore, the extensive behavior observations we are recommending are expensive, time consuming, and in some cases *reactive.* (Reactive measures are those that interfere with the behavior they are intended to measure. See Lana, 1969; Webb, Campbell, Schwartz, and Sechrest, 1966.) We welcome the development of technologies that would allow us to make better use of our time. Unfortunately, the most promising technologies – such as electromechanical devices (see Schwitzgebel and Schwitzgebel, 1973), videotaping, and standardized tests – either are not yet sufficiently refined to provide the specific information required or are not yet produced inexpensively enough to be readily available for student projects.

Overview

We hope that an efficient and reliable data collection method will be a basic feature of your experimental behavior modification project. This method should provide data on the target behavior(s) throughout the various stages or conditions of your project: first during the baseline condition that occurs prior to any formal treatment intervention* and thereafter during treatment and control conditions as well as during follow-up.

A comparison of baseline rates of the target behavior with rates obtained during and following treatment will allow you to determine whether your child-client has improved; other comparisons will assist you in assessing the durability and generality of the change as well as whether the change can be attributed to the specific techniques you employed (A more extensive discussion of methods for identifying the effective therapeutic ingredient is presented in the following chapter on experimental control.)

The generally accepted steps to be followed in developing an effective method of data collection (see, for example, Bijou et al., 1968; Johnston and Harris, 1968; Wright, 1967) include the following:

1. Define the target behavior(s) in a way suitable for measurement.
2. Develop a measuring device.
3. Decide when to take data.
4. Determine the context of observations.
5. Assess reliability and observer bias.

It is the purpose of this chapter to provide a detailed description of how each of steps one through four can be successfully accomplished; reliability will be discussed in Chapter 7. You may find some of the tasks we suggest time

*One must be wary of referring to the baseline condition as a no-treatment condition. Duncan (1969, p. 545) quotes Lindsley as saying that in 5% of the 2000 cases on file with him behaviors changed solely in response to having had those behaviors observed and recorded.

consuming and even tedious. We believe, however, that the added information provided by good data makes the effort well worthwhile.

DEFINE THE TARGET BEHAVIOR

Once you have selected a target behavior, define it in a way suitable for measurement. As Chapter 2 pointed out, one cannot safely assume that the caretaker's initial description of the target behavior will be satisfactory. Your aim is to achieve a response definition that is meaningful, behavioral, and that produces reliable data.

Meaningful, as used here, resembles the term *valid,* as used in the test and measurement literature. While there are many different conceptions and methods of validation, as Campbell and Fiske (1959, p.81) point out, "validation is typically convergent." Thus, your response definition should converge or generally agree with the target response as defined by the child's caretakers; if possible, it should be consistent with the definition used in related behavior change projects. While concerns with validity have not been prominent in the writings of behavior modifiers, the importance of validity issues is highlighted in a recent important paper by Johnson and Bolstad (1973, pp. 50-58).

In order for your definition to be behavioral, it should be described in terms of *specific observable responses.* You have already had experience in making narrative accounts of your child-client's observable behavior in naturalistic situations, and you are aware of the pitfalls of making inferences about intent, internal states, and other private events. Apply the same precautions when you define the target behavior(s).

The final characteristic of a good definition is that it produces reliable data. Reliability in this context refers to the degree to which *independent observers agree* on the occurrence and nonoccurrence of the target response. According to Gellert (1955, p. 194): "the fewer the categories, the more precise their definition, and the less inference required in making classifications, the greater will be the reliability of the data." Campbell (1961, p. 340) adds: "The greater the direct accessibility of the stimuli to sense receptors, the greater the intersubjective verifiability of the observation. The weaker or the more intangible, indirect, or abstract the stimulus attribute, the more the observations are subject to distortion." Thus, for example, it is easy to measure eating in terms of number of forkfulls a child places in his mouth, but difficult to count the number of chewing movements he makes. It is easier to count math problems completed than it is to monitor eye contact or verbal behavior. Try to define target responses in such a way that they can be easily and reliably measured.

Remember, most target responses can be defined in a variety of ways. A target behavior such as aggression-toward-teacher could be defined in terms of (a) the number of bites, scratches, and hits, (b) the amount of time spent biting, scratching, and hitting, or (c) the intensity of the bites, scratches, and hits. These are all *direct* measures of aggression. Another tactic that may work is to measure the number of bandaids applied to the victimized teacher. This is an *indirect* measure, and its acceptability as a measure of aggression must be demonstrated by showing its relationship to a direct measure. For example, the teacher may apply a bandaid each time little Timmy has drawn blood – a direct measure; so there is a reliable relationship between depth of abrasion and bandaid application.

Topographic vs. Functional Definitions

There are two general approaches to defining and describing target behaviors (Hutt and Hutt, 1970). The first approach is to define a response in terms of its *topography*, or the movements comprising the response. The second approach is to define a response in terms of its *function*, or the effects it has on the environment. Consider the examples of thumb-sucking and window-breaking. Thumb-sucking would be defined topographically, for example, as the child's having his thumb or any other finger touching or between his lips or fully inserted into his mouth between his teeth. This definition informs recorders that the child's having his thumb to his chin or near his mouth does not constitute thumb-sucking. Any disagreement between observers might then be due to failure to observe accurately rather than to disagreement on definitions.

Window-breaking, on the other hand, would be defined functionally, and the definition would focus on what constitutes a broken window. The definition need not specify the precise movements or responses required to break a window – a task that might prove difficult when working with an inventive and persistent child-client.

Which of these two definitional approaches you take will depend largely on the nature of your target behavior. As Hutt and Hutt (p. 33) indicate, "some behavioral abnormalities are manifested primarily in the morphological (topographical) characteristics of behavior, and others by the specificity of the changes wrought upon the environment." Still other problem behaviors require specification of both topography and function, as, for example, the definition of "bullying" given in Table 3-1.

Table 3-1 A Sample Definition (Bullying) Including Both Topographic and Functional Elements

Antecedent Event	Topographical Description	Functional Description
Victim nearby	Hit, kick; bite; scratch; pull hair or clothing	Victim cries and/or runs away (within 30")

Questionable instances. With behaviors that present definition difficulties, it is often a good idea to develop a list of questionable responses and then decide that "tooth-picking with lips parted" might not constitute a recordable instance of thumb-sucking, whereas "a knuckle touching or between the lips or fully inserted into the mouth between the teeth" would constitute a positive or scorable response. The more scoring examples you can present to your observers, the higher your agreement regarding response definitions is likely to be. The definition and scorable and unscorable examples might be prepared in a manner similar to the material presented in Table 3-2. If decisions about novel questionable responses must be made after data collection has begun, note your decisions in some convenient and accessible place, such as an observer's logbook or on the data sheet itself.

Table 3-2 A Sample Definition with Scorable and Unscorable Instances of Peer Interaction

Definition of Peer Interaction:	Peer interaction is scored when the child is (a) within three feet of a peer and either (b) engaged in conversation or physical activity with the peer or (c) jointly using a toy or other play object.
Instances:	"Gimme a cookie" directed at tablemate; Hitting another child; Walking hand-in-hand; Sharing a jar of paint; Waiting for a turn in a group play activity.
Noninstances:	Not interacting while standing in line; Two children independently but concurrently talking to a teacher.

Additional information on response definitions can be found in a number of sources, including Ayllon and Azrin (1968, Chapter 3), Bijou et al. (1968), Hutt and Hutt (1970), and Wright (1967).

Probe Questions for Part 1, Chapter 3

1. It is sometimes argued that data collection requires more time and effort than it is worth. What are the primary advantages and disadvantages of data collection?

2. If target behaviors for modification programs are typically identified by parents or teachers, why shouldn't we accept their descriptions (or definitions) of the troublesome behaviors without change?

3. Describe and explain the requirements of a good target response definition.

4. Why might one *not* wish to define "appropriate care of pets" in terms of the longevity of the family goldfish?

5. Why is it usually a good practice to accompany a definition with instances and noninstances?

6. What is a topographic definition? What is a functional definition?

Behavioral Objectives for Part 2, Chapter 3

After studying Part 2 of this chapter, you should be able to:

1. Select an appropriate response characteristic for measurement, such as frequency or duration.

2. Decide upon a level of quantification suitable for your target behavior.

3. Select an appropriate response-recording technique.

4. Determine whether the tally, duration, or interval method is appropriate for your study.

5. Develop behavior codes and design useful data sheets.

Part 2. Developing a Measuring Procedure

We have available to us an extremely wide variety of methods of obtaining response data – an observation familiar to those who have completed courses in experimental psychology. Finding one's way through the thicket of alternatives requires attention to three questions: First, what characteristic of the response should be measured? Second, what level of measurement should be employed? And third, what kind of recording procedure should be used?

Select the Appropriate Response Characteristic

Some responses, such as problem-solving, are best measured in terms of frequency; others, such as crying, are better measured in terms of duration; still others are better measured in terms of latency (responsiveness to requests), volume (amount of milk drunk), amplitude (loudness of screams), or extension (distance crawled). The definition you developed in the previous section will probably limit the response characteristics appropriate for inclusion in your study. Practical considerations, such as requirements of time and the availability of suitable measuring instruments, will further narrow the alternatives.

Consider a response such as napping. Napping would not ordinarily be measured in terms of volume, extension, or amplitude. But the frequency of naps, their latency (time taken to fall asleep), or duration (time slept) might be suitable characteristics to measure. The frequency or number of naps may be the easiest of the three characteristics to measure, but before you choose it be sure that it will be sensitive to your treatment manipulations. When frequency is the characteristic of naps measured, a one-minute nap may be equivalent to a three-hour nap. So you may wish to choose an alternative characteristic to measure nap-taking.

Select a Level of Measurement

Once you have decided which response characteristics to measure, you must decide what level of measurement to use. Assume that our target behavior was spilling food and we were trying to decrease it. The response characteristic of interest was amount of spilling. The most precise measure of amount of spilling might be obtained by weighing the child and the food on his plate before the meal and again after the meal. The preweight minus the postweight would then give a *quantitative, continuous* measure of the amount (weight) of food spilled. If spilling had been restricted to the tablecloth, we might count the number of soiled spots. This would provide a *quantitative, discrete* (only integer values allowed) measure of the amount of food spilled. We still have additional alternatives. We could determine for each meal if spilling occurred or not. This would provide a *dichotomous* (two category), *discrete* measure of spilling. Additional examples could be developed for this problem; however, the important point to note is that each successive example was cruder in terms of measurement than the prior examples. That is, the earlier examples included more information and allowed for finer discriminations. This increased precision has a drawback, however; generally, the more precise the measurement, the more expensive (e.g., time consuming) it is to obtain.

It is important, then, in deciding upon a useful level of measurement to balance the two factors of precision and expense. The measure must be precise enough to show changes in the target behavior, but inexpensive enough not to be a burden on you, the child, or his caretakers. In the example of spilling described above, the first measure that involved weighing of the child might be quite inconvenient, whereas the measure of spilling that required a yes-no response to each meal might not be sensitive to changes in the child's eating behavior. You may, for example, reduce spilling from 15 times per meal to once per meal, but the dichotomous measure of spilling would not reflect this change.

Select a Recording Technique

After you have decided what to observe and how to observe it, you must then decide what kind of recording technique to use. If your target response leaves a record (such as soiled diapers, an unmade bed, or a written answer), you are in luck; all you need do is examine the record and tabulate the response.* In addition, you need not worry about the reactive effects that human observers sometimes have on the target behavior! A number of intriguing examples of trace or record-leaving responses can be found in Webb et al. (1966).

*At times, the processes intervening between examining the record and tabulating the response are somewhat more complicated. For example, assume the target behavior was writing one's name legibly. A judgment, perhaps a complex judgment, would have to be made of the product to determine whether or the degree to which the written product achieved the intelligibility criterion. This, in turn, might require periodic independent ratings (or rankings) by an independent judge. Methods of arriving at qualitative assessments of behavioral products are described in Cronbach (1970, Chapter 17). Examples of how such complex judgments can be made reliably are found in Goetz and Baer (1973) and in Hopkins, Schutte, and Garton (1971).

If, instead, your target behavior is ephemeral and leaves no record, the recording techniques most frequently used require a clipboard, stopwatch and data sheets of one type or another, and of course a human observer. The following sections describe the three methods most commonly used with human observers: the tally, duration, and interval methods.

Tally method. For many behaviors, the easiest method of gathering data is simply to count or tally the number of occurrences of the behavior, as you have defined it, in some predetermined time interval. For example, the tally method might be used in observing a young child who has an inappropriately high rate of squealing. You would count each time the child squeals during a specified time interval, such as 9:00 to 11:30 a.m., or within each of 30 five-minute time intervals spread throughout the school day. The latter method might be preferable because of the more representative data it provides.

In applied behavioral work with children, the tally method has been used with a variety of discrete behaviors, such as instruction-following (Whitman, Zakaras, and Chardos, 1971), language usage (Schumaker and Sherman, 1970), and vomiting (Wolf, Birnbrauer, Williams, and Lawler, 1965). The tally method has also been used to track multiple behaviors in a single child (Lovaas and Simmons, 1969). This complex recording task is most easily done with sophisticated keyboards and event recorders (see Lovaas, Freitag, Gold, and Kassorla, 1965). Additional information on the tally method can be found in Bijou et al. (1968), Herbert (1970), and in recent issues of *Behavior Therapy* and the *Journal of Applied Behavior Analysis.*

Duration method. This method is used in cases in which the duration of the behavior rather than its daily frequency is the essential feature. To use the duration method, run a stopwatch continuously while the behavior is occurring during an observation period of a specified length. An example of the use of this method would be recording the amount of time a child sucks his thumb. While the child sucks his thumb, the watch is running; when he stops sucking, the watch is stopped. To get adequate duration data, use a watch to time the total duration of the observation session and a stopwatch to record duration of the target behavior.

O'Brien, Azrin, and Bugle (1972) used the duration method, as well as the tally method, to chart changes in a child's locomotion from crawling to walking as a result of their training procedures. The duration method also has been used successfully in measuring changes in thumb-sucking as a function of the contingent reinforcement of incompatible responses (Skiba, Pettigrew, and Alden, 1971). While these two studies represent only a fraction of those studies using the duration method, it is apparent that this is the least used of the three common response measures. We suspect that this is due in part to the belief that frequency is a more basic response characteristic (Bijou et al.,

1969; Skinner, 1966) and in part to the greater efficiency of estimating duration by the interval method, which is discussed below.

Note: If you decide that either the tally or duration method is appropriate for your study, the daily observation period (say 20 minutes) should be divided into eight to 12 intervals of *equal* length for purposes of reliability assessment. The necessity for doing so will become apparent in the chapter on reliability (Chapter 7).

Interval method. To use the interval method of recording, break the observation period into small *equal* intervals and record whether or not the behavior is observed to occur in each interval. The interval size will usually be from five seconds to one minute in duration, depending upon (a) the rate of the response and (b) the average duration of a single response. For high-rate behaviors, the interval should be sufficiently small so that two complete responses could not occur in a single interval. On the other hand, the interval should be at least as long as the average duration of a single response. The use of excessively long intervals would obviously result in an underestimate of the occurrence frequency of the target behavior, and might result in your underestimation of the size of the reduction of an undesirable behavior as a result of a deceleration program. The use of very small intervals would have the opposite effect.

Interval-recording techniques, because they provide close approximation to either frequency or duration recording of target behaviors, are applicable to a variety of target behaviors, so you may find them useful in your project. The interval method has been used to record changes in mealtime behavior (Barton, Guess, Garcia, and Baer, 1970), studying (Hall, Lund, and Jackson, 1968), attending (Walker and Buckley, 1968), talking (Reynolds and Risley, 1968), playing (Buell, Stoddard, Harris, and Baer, 1968), and disruptive behaviors (O'Leary, Becker, Evans, and Saudargas, 1969). For further details on the specific interval-recording technique employed, refer to the papers cited.

With the interval-recording method, as with any of the other methods, you must adopt consistent rules on when to record behavior. The rule must be *either* (a) behavior is counted as occurring on the basis of the proportion of the interval during which it took place, e.g., 50 per cent or more of the interval to be rated as occurring, or (b) whether behavior occurred at any time during the interval. Otherwise you may get fluctuating standards for rating occurrences and consequent lowered interrater agreement. Of these two rules governing rating the occurrence of a behavior, the latter requires less judgment and is perhaps the easier procedure to employ, although it may give an overestimate of absolute frequency or duration of the target behavior.

If your intervals are short and you are observing more than one behavior, you might find that your reliability is lowered because you and your fellow observer are not coordinating your observing and tabulating time. If this is a problem, you might try a slight variation of these procedures; use one interval for observing and the next for recording. Or, if the intervals are longer, (say 20 seconds), the first 15 seconds might be used for observing and the final five seconds for recording. The use of a strategy such as this might substantially improve the quality of your data.

If you intend to use time intervals shorter than 30 seconds, you will find it necessary to develop some signaling device that alerts you to the end of one interval and the beginning of the next. We have found the use of a portable cassette audio tape recorder to be an efficient and unobtrusive means of signaling observation and recording intervals. To use the recorder, first prepare a tape on which you speak the number of each observation and recording interval. A tape so constructed might begin with "Interval 1, observe" (ten seconds of silence or whatever the length of your observation interval, "Interval 1, record" (five seconds of silence or whatever the time required to record your observations), "Interval 2, observe," etc. Then, while you make the behavior observations, carry the tape recorder and use an ear-piece speaker to listen to the prerecorded interval signals. If the intervals on your recording sheets are similarly numbered, you need not worry about tabulating your entries in the wrong recording interval. Another useful signaling device – an electronic tone generator with adjustable time intervals – is described by Worthy (1968). Both of these methods allow you to observe the child without the distractions necessitated by having to keep track of the time with a watch. But the use of recorded numbers that identify the recording interval produce clearly superior reliability when compared with a tone or beep that does not identify the recording interval (Whelan, 1974).

The flow chart* shown in Fig. 3-1 will help you decide which recording method is most suitable for your project. To use this chart, begin at the upper left-hand corner and answer each successive question until you reach the appropriate recording method. If you have had considerable experience as an observer, you may prefer to use a method somewhat different from those indicated in the flow chart. For example, when you are observing more than one behavior or subject at a time, it may be more convenient for you to use the tally method than the interval method. (See papers by Bijou et al. [1968], Boer [1968], and Schaeffer and Martin [1969] for descriptions of sampling procedures typically used when observing more than one child.)

*This flow chart is based on material presented by Jackson, Della-Piana, and Sloane (1971) and by Alevizos, Campbell, Callahan, and Berck (1974).

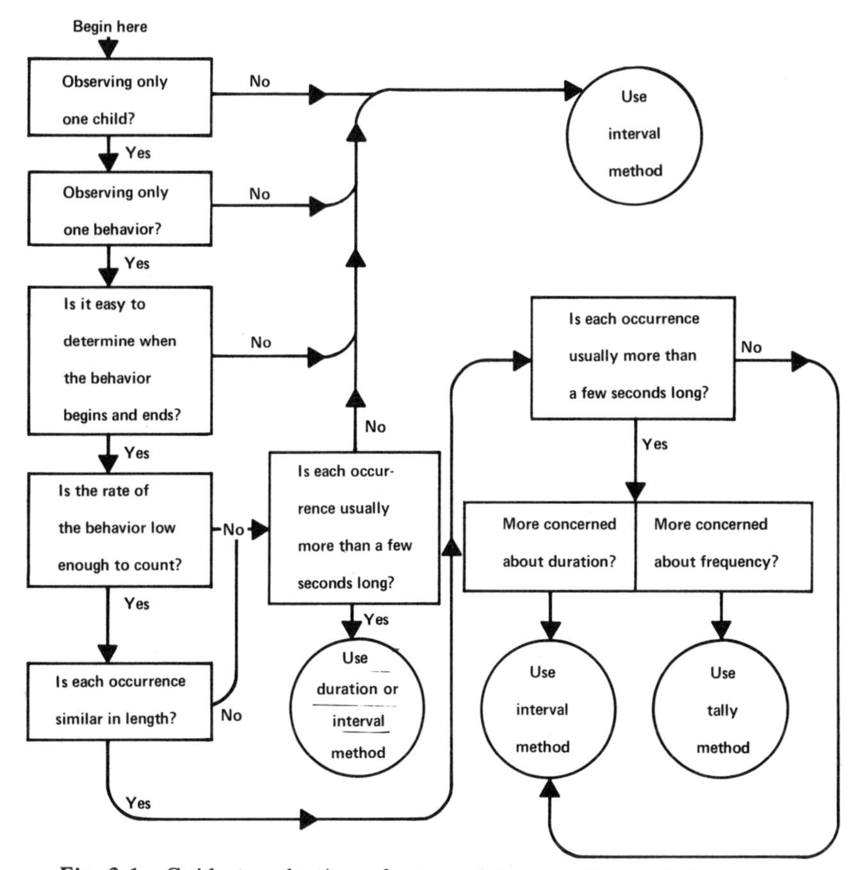

Fig. 3-1. Guide to selection of appropriate recording technique.

Whatever recording device you use, be sure that it is in good working order. With human observers, this implies – among other things – that you should attend to elementary rules of human engineering. For example, the use of behavioral codes and well-constructed data sheets may make the difference between confusing uninterpretable data and useful data. Similarly, attention to such seemingly trivial details as availability of clipboards with attached pencils and coordination of stopwatches can spare you from data loss and unexplainable poor reliability.

Develop behavioral codes. Develop a coding system to save observer writing and recording time. If a single target behavior is being recorded, a simple tally mark or activation of a wrist golf-score counter can be used to indicate each occurrence. If several behaviors are being studied, a single-letter abbreviation for each behavior is useful – e.g., P to indicate play behavior. Keep the code simple by minimizing the number of pencil strokes required for each tally, by using a unique and easily discriminated symbol for each behavior, and by using symbols that remind you of the behaviors they signify – e.g., use V for smiles and Λ for frowns. That way the symbols won't be confused. Helpful information on behavioral codes can be found in Bijou et al. (1968), in Johnston and Harris (1968), and in Patterson, Ray, Shaw, and Cobb (1969).

Design and duplicate data sheets. A well-designed data sheet is an indispensable part of a high quality data collection method. A sample data sheet is shown in Table 3-3. Be certain to date each data sheet and indicate the time and situation, including the names of other people who may be present. If more than one child or more than one behavior is being observed, also indicate the appropriate additional names and behavior codes. Nothing is quite so discouraging as concluding a study and finding a set of unlabeled (hence uninterpretable) data sheets. You should also *number the recording intervals,* as this will insure correspondence between the intervals indicated by the signaling device and the interval to be used on the data sheet. It will also facilitate data retrieval and comparison of data following reliability checks. Don't forget to include a "comments" section on the data sheet. Use this space for noting hunches about possible controlling variables, noteworthy therapist behaviors, and any irregularities that might affect the results.

Table 3-3 Sample Data Sheet

Date ______ Session number ______ Child ____________ Therapist __________

Time started ______ Time concluded ______ Observer ____________________

Setting: (e.g., tutoring booth, classroom, family dining room) ______________

Activity ____

BEHAVIOR CODES: (e.g., I = interactive play
S = solitary play)

1	2	3	4	5	6	7	8	9	10	11	12	13	14	15

16	17	18	19	20	21	22	23	24	25	26	27	28	29	30

31	32	33	34	35	36	37	38	39	40	41	42	43	44	45

46	47	48	49	50	51	52	53	54	55	56	57	58	59	60

61	62	63	64	65	66	67	68	69	70	71	72	73	74	75

76	77	78	79	80	81	82	83	84	85	86	87	88	89	90

91	92	93	94	95	96	97	98	99	100	101	102	103	104	105

106	107	108	109	110	111	112	113	114	115	116	117	118	119	120

Comments: (Include descriptions of unusual events, indications of child's ill health, competing activities, etc., that might have an impact on the child's behavior.)

Probe Questions for Part 2, Chapter 3

1. The target behavior to be increased in rate is napping. Which response characteristic (e.g., volume, color, pitch, amplitude) might be most appropriate for measurement purposes?

2. What is the tally method and when might you want to use it?

3. Which of the three methods of taking observational data (e.g., tally, duration, and interval) has the widest applicability? Why?

4. Tom's mother has defined "picking-up clothes" as the target behavior for an acceleration program. She has a number of options available for measuring the amount of clothing not picked up, including weighing them, counting them, and simply indicating whether or not all the clothing has been picked up. What kind of measurement does each procedure provide? What are their advantages and disadvantages?

5. What are the characteristics of a good behavior code?

6. Give examples of trace or record-leaving behaviors and of ephemeral behaviors.

7. Say that you want to record whether a child is playing alone, interacting with peers, or interacting with teachers, and whether peers or teachers attend to his approach attempts. Select a simple, easily discriminated code symbol for each of these five events.

Behavioral Objectives for Part 3, Chapter 3

When you have read Part 3 of this chapter, you should be able to:

1. Determine when to collect data on the target behavior during your study.

2. Distinguish between free and discriminated operants.

3. Distinguish between time sampling and event sampling.

4. Describe the advantages of data probes.

5. Distinguish between the various kinds of generalization that have relevance to a treatment study.

Part 3. Determining the Time and Context of Data Collection

In a broad sense, the answer to the question "when to collect data" has already been given: during the baseline, treatment, and control conditions, and, if possible, some time (perhaps two weeks to a month) following the termination of the last treatment phase. A week of data collection during this follow-up period is a small cost to pay for information on the durability of the behavior change you produced, and it is usually worthwhile.

Given that data should be collected during each of these various phases, a problem still remains concerning when during these phases of your study the data should be collected. Unfortunately, there are few useful generalizations that can be given to this question. You might think that an ideal answer is "all the time," but this may not be the case. Consider, for example, the target behavior setting-the-table. It would be foolhardy to collect data on that behavior at times other than at mealtimes. It would be equally inefficient to collect data on the target behavior of saying "Good morning, teacher" at a place other than school and at a time other than the morning.

You must decide when to schedule observation periods and when during the observation periods to collect data. At one extreme the entire day could constitute the observation period, while at the other extreme a small segment of the day (such as lunch time) could constitute the period of data collection. Within the selected observation period, data could be collected *continuously* or *sampled* on some basis during that period of time. Your decision on when to collect data hinges on (a) the nature of the target behavior, (b) the nature of your treatment interventions, (c) the purpose of your study, and finally (d) various practical considerations such as the amount of observer time available and the extent and regularity of your access to the child-client.

Nature of the target response. A method of classifying target responses that is useful in determining when data should be collected is the extent to which the behavior is under specific and known stimulus control. At one extreme are behaviors (such as walking, thumb-sucking, and crying) that are not under tight stimulus control; they occur almost any time and any number of times. These responses, if they are under the control of consequences, are called *free operants.* Free operants can be measured either continuously (sometimes referred to as *event sampling*) or by means of a *time-sampling* procedure. Consider the target behavior of crying. A caretaker, almost certainly a parent or staff member of an institution, could stay near at hand with a stopwatch, clicking the watch on and off with the beginning and end of each crying episode for 24 hours of a child's day. Or, instead, crying might be measured by noting whether it occurred during each hourly strike of a clock chime or an oven timer. This latter method is referred to as time sampling. For an excellent review of time-sampling procedures, see Arrington (1943).

On the other extreme of the continuum are behaviors that ordinarily occur only under highly limited stimulus conditions. These *discriminated* operants include responses such as appropriate eating behavior, fighting with siblings, and leaving the bed during naptime. These responses may vary in rate, but they occur only in specific stimulus situations. Consequently, it makes little sense to observe these behaviors continuously throughout the day. They may, however, be observed continuously throughout the situation in which they occur. Data could be taken throughout mealtime, or naptime, or, in the case of sibling aggression, whenever a sibling is present. Alternatively, data could be sampled within these occasions. For example, the child could be observed every five minutes during his three meals and data taken on the proportion of time during which he was engaged in "pigging" (Barton et al., 1970).

A subclass of discriminated operants is sometimes referred to as *discrete trial responses.* In discrete trial responding, only a single response can be given to each presentation of a specific stimulus; for example, catching or not catching a ball when it is thrown, compliance or noncompliance to a request such as "Close the door," greeting relatives when they enter the house, and flushing the toilet after using it. It should be obvious that data on discrete trial responses should be taken only when a trial occurs. Again, data could be gathered during each trial or only sampled on some trials.

Sampling of discrete trials, particularly during a training session, is sometimes called a *data probe.* Probing has much to recommend it in contrast to taking data continuously during a training session – a task that is best performed by either an observer or by a practiced trainer with unusual dexterity. Consider a training session in which you are training a child to say "baby" (or to swim, throw a ball, or solve long-division problems). The specific techniques you use during a training session might include prompting, modeling, guided participation, in addition to various consequating procedures (see Chapter 5). To attempt to tabulate only the child's responses into categories of no-response, partially correct response, prompted response, and correct response while managing both the stimuli and the consequences would be an almost unmanageable feat. Contrast this with the relative ease of probing the child's responses – perhaps at the beginning and end of the session – by noting how he responds to three unreinforced presentations of the instruction, "Say 'baby'." Unless you can conveniently use continuous data collection techniques during training, use probes.

Nature of the intervention procedures. At one extreme, your intervention procedures might be in effect throughout the child's entire day, such as might be the case if you were trying to train toileting behaviors in a young child. At the other extreme, treatment might only be applied for a very limited part of a child's day, as would be the case if the target behavior were swimming or table manners.

In the case of behaviors trained throughout the day, data might be either sampled or gathered continuously throughout the day. In the case of more discrete training programs, data again could be obtained continuously or sampled (probed), but during the occasions when training is taking place.

Purposes of the study. If the purpose of your study is only to demonstrate that a response has been changed in a highly specific situation (such as a one-half hour training session), then all you need do is collect data during that training session. If, instead, your horizons are broader and you want to assert that the change has greater *generality,* you must collect additional data. (See Chapter 9 for a discussion of the advisability of including generalization training in your treatment program.)

Before examining what types of additional data need to be collected and where, a number of types of generalization should be distinguished. First, one might be interested in insuring that the response is maintained when other people function as trainers (trainer generalization), in other training situations (situational generalization), or in response to other training stimuli (stimulus generalization or concept formation). The latter type of generalization would be demonstrated if, after a child correctly labeled as blue a blue ball (the training stimulus), he also correctly labeled as blue the sky, a blue shirt, and a blue truck.

Obviously, the data collection requirements of these various forms of generalization differ. In the first case (trainer generalization), additional generalization sessions would be conducted in which a different person performed the role of trainer. Situational generalization requires conducting sessions in a different situation (e.g., another room), while stimulus generalization requires probing the child on additional test stimuli – perhaps during the regular training session. The latter measurements are sometimes referred to as *generalization probes.*

Let us examine more closely an example of situational generality. Assume, for example, that training was directed at increasing a child's "attention span" for two daily 20-minute sessions and that changes were observed during those sessions. It may not be true, however, that the child's "attention span" had changed during other periods of time. (It is entirely acceptable and well within the tradition of much behavior modification work with children to observe the target behavior only during training sessions. However, the change has much greater social relevance if it also occurs outside of the training session, and observations taken outside of the session may be worth the brief time required.) In order to conclude that the target behavior has generalized broadly, data must be obtained either continuously throughout the day (which is difficult at best) or from representatively sampled occasions. Less broad but nonetheless useful conclusions about generalization can be made by observing the target behavior in but one extratreatment situation in which it is likely to occur. For example, instruction-following, trained in a limited treatment setting, could also be observed at home during a time when instructions are regularly given.

Convenience. The last consideration, convenience, requires little amplification. If data are to be gathered by human observers (rather than by electronic or mechanical devices), convenience for the observers is a crucial determinant of the amount of data that can be obtained. Continuous data obviously cannot be gathered throughout the day unless the child is young and a member of one's own family; data can be sampled only at those times when the child is available. Complex data can only be obtained when an independent observer is present. You should carefully consider the practical demands placed on the data collector; unreasonable demands will probably result in disgruntled, demoralized observers and poor quality data. Table 3-4 presents some general rules that you may find useful in deciding when and how often to collect data.

Table 3-4 General Rules for When and How Often to Collect Data

A.	If your treatment intervention occurs during a brief training session, but it is desirable that the behavior occur in other situations:	
	DO	take data during the training session.
	DO NOT	attempt to take *continuous* data during the training session if you are both trainer and observer; instead use data *probes.*
	DO	include *generalization probes* if at all possible.
B.	If the target behavior is a discriminated operant:	
	DO	take data in the stimulus condition in which the behavior occurs.
	DO NOT	take data at random periods throughout the day.
C.	If the target behavior is a free operant:	
	DO	take data at random periods throughout the day.
	DO NOT	use a few long observation periods if you are able to use many short observation periods.

D. And, finally, whatever the nature of the target response:
DO NOT make unreasonable demands on the observers (or on the child and his caretakers).

If during data collection you are a classroom or home visitor, or if your presence as an observer represents a novel situation for the child, some added precautions are warranted. First, the child will probably react to your presence. Consequently, the first few days of observation may be unrepresentative of the child's natural behavior and probably should be discarded. (That's just as well because the method you use during your first few days of data collection will most probably require modification.) In order to reduce the effects of the observer on the data, review and follow the guidelines for observer conduct offered in Part 3 of Chapter 2.

Finally, you should make some tentative decision about what should be done in the event of unforeseen interruptions or other distracting events. Will you continue to record data, move the child to another room, discontinue data collection for a short period, or terminate the day's observation session? Not all untoward events can be foreseen, but those that can should be planned for.

This concludes our discussion of the basic development of a data collection method. Many of the issues are perhaps even more complicated than we have indicated. If you are interested in gaining more information on these topics, you may want to examine Arrington (1939, 1943), Boyd and DeVault (1966), Gellert (1955), Heyns and Lippitt (1954), Hutt and Hutt (1970), Kerlinger (1964, Chapter 28), Weick (1968), or Wright (1960).

Probe Questions for Part 3, Chapter 3

1. Alternative methods of data collection are being discussed as part of a program to teach shoe-tying. Would this behavior be considered a free operant? If a sampling method were to be used, would it be a time-sampling or event-sampling method?

2. What do the responses of catching a ball, responding to a request, and closing a door all have in common?

3. What factors should be considered in determining when to collect data?

4. What rules of conduct should be observed when observing children in either a home or school setting?

5. What are the primary advantages of using data probes?

6. You are requiring a reluctant observer to travel to a child's home on Sunday evening to record the child's completion of homework assignments. What are the probable effects on the observer's behavior and the data collected? What other methods might be used to collect the same data?

Behavioral Objectives for Part 1, Chapter 4

After studying Part 1 of this chapter, you should be able to:

1. State the major purpose of demonstrating experimental control.

2. State the major threats to internal validity and guard against them in your study.

CHAPTER 4

Demonstration of Experimental Control

Part 1. Introduction and Threats to Internal Validity

INTRODUCTION

Up to this point in your treatment program, you have set up appropriate contacts with the child's caretakers, completed a detailed behavior assessment (including narrative observations of the child in his natural environment and discussions with the child and his caretakers), and perhaps selected a tentative treatment strategy. Before beginning your program, you should study this and the preceding chapter on developing a data collection system, as they provide the backbone for the scientific portion of your study.

Any mention of experimental design recalls for some students their boredom associated with learning about rats in mazes and college sophomores' responses to endlessly turning memory drums. For some, the mention of data and the numbers used to represent them can precipitate an anxiety attack. But take heart. We have tried to minimize these effects – first by directing our discussion of experimental designs to those directly relevant to your work with children, and second, wherever possible, by avoiding esoteric, statistically related terms. The closest we come to things statistical in this section is the binocular test, and you already have the equipment for that.

We hope that you integrate the material in this and the following chapter into your project; your failure to do so will simply result in one more uncontrolled case study in behavior modification (Pawlicki, 1970). If, on the other hand, you do include this material, your study will qualify as an experiment in the best sense of that term.

There are several interdependent questions that you will want to consider in evaluating your project.

1. Did your target behavior's rate change reliably during the study? In order to answer this question, the target behavior must be carefully defined and reliably measured during the course of the study. A functional presentation of the material on definitions, reliability, and methods of developing continuous data procedures is given in the preceding and the following chapters.

2. If reliable changes in the target behavior have occurred, can these changes be attributed to your treatment procedures (those child management changes that occurred between baseline and treatment)?

3. Finally, if the changes can be attributed to your treatment procedures, can you specify unequivocally which of the child management techniques was the effective change ingredient?

If you are able to answer either of the latter two questions affirmatively, and we think you will, you will have achieved a fundamental goal of science – that is, you will have established a cause-effect relationship between variables. In your case the cause-effect relationship will be between a child behavior – the target behavior – and an intervention technique or set of techniques.

The methods of demonstrating cause-effect relationships are discussed in texts on experimental design by Campbell and Stanley (1963), D'Amato (1970), Underwood (1957), and others. Unfortunately, these and most other experimental design texts used by students in their undergraduate curriculum focus on tactics of experimental design for group research. Certainly the principles of good design are the same whether one is studying groups of subjects or a single subject. However, the specific application of these principles to the design of single subject (N=1) studies is sufficiently different to warrant a somewhat detailed presentation of this material. Before providing information to aid you in selecting an experimental design appropriate for your study, we will examine the factors that must be controlled if you are to be confident that your treatment effects are genuine and your cause-effect statements accurate.

THREATS TO INTERNAL VALIDITY

A good experimental design should protect against the major threats to internal validity. These threats are simply extraneous factors or confounding variables which, if not controlled, might be mistaken for a treatment effect. Those factors that threaten the internal validity of N=1 studies include the following (Campbell and Stanley, 1963, p. 5):

1. History – the specific events, such as illnesses and changes of school, occurring to the child between baseline and follow-up in addition to treatment.

2. Maturation – processes within the child operating as a function of time; e.g., "growing out of" a problem because of increased size, weight, or coordination.

3. Testing – the effects of an initial measurement upon subsequent measurements; e.g., "I'm being observed again so I had better shape up. The last time I was observed I goofed off and then had to sit in a room every afternoon and eat M&M's."

4. Instrumentation – changes in the calibration of observers that produce changes in the obtained measurements (i.e., instrument decay). For example, the criteria for a scorable response may change throughout the study. Consequently, lower rates of undesirable behavior observed at the end of the study are due not to changes in the child but to changes in the response definition.

5. Statistical regression – a phenomenon in which a child selected because of his deviancy will score less deviantly upon further measurement.

Consider how these five threats to internal validity might operate in a traditional, but weak, experimental design for evaluating change in a single subject. The design could be diagrammed as O X O, where the O's represent pre- and postmeasures and X is the treatment. Assume that the problem behavior was sibling aggression and that the rate of aggression decreased between the pretest and posttest. Can we safely attribute this change to treatment? Definitely not! Lower rates of aggression could be due to some environmental event (i.e., history) that occurred at approximately the same time but independently of treatment – for example, the visit of a doting grandparent, or the departure of a troublesome sibling for summer camp. Perhaps the child has undergone a growth spurt (maturation) coincidentally with treatment, so that an older brother is no longer physically superior and consequently no longer instigates the child-client. Perhaps the initial measurement of peer aggression sensitized the child to his own aggressive behavior, and this alone resulted in lower rates of aggression on the posttest (testing). Perhaps the observer, who might also have been the therapist, developed a more stringent definition of aggression at the time of the second testing (instrumentation); that such calibration changes in observers are possible is suggested by the work of Rosenthal (1966) on experimental bias. Finally, perhaps the child's initial rate of aggressive behavior during the pretest was the highest rate he had ever displayed. If his selection for treatment was based on that high rate, the posttest rate would almost certainly decrease (regression).

In order to avoid mistaking these five factors for a treatment effect, it will be necessary for you to include additional experimental design features over and above the O X O features of the design described above. Be alert, because the features will generally differ from those to which you have been exposed in experimental design classes that focused on group research.

Probe Questions for Part 1, Chapter 4

1. What are the questions that should be answered by a good experimental design?

2. What are the five primary threats to internal validity?

3. Why would a change in classroom teacher that occurred coincidentally with treatment present an interpretation problem?

4. What are regression effects?

Behavioral Objectives for Part 2, Chapter 4

After reading Part 2 of this chapter, you should be able to:

1. State the defining characteristics of the reversal or ABAB procedure and the advantages and limitations of this design.

2. State the type of problem behaviors for which the ABAB design is most appropriate.

Part 2. Within-Subject Designs: The Reversal Design

WITHIN-SUBJECT (N=1) DESIGNS

There are two general families of experimental designs that might be employed in demonstrating control with a single subject. The first and most common is called an ABAB design or a reversal design. The second design type is a time-lagged multiple time series – more simply, a multiple baseline procedure. Introductions to these designs are given by Baer et al. (1968). Sidman (1960) presents a detailed rationale and discussion of their application to experimentation with animals.

Our discussions of these designs will primarily be directed to answering the second question posed at the beginning of the chapter: Are the intervention technique(s) I employed responsible for the changes in the child's target behavior? For certain simple intervention strategies, a straightforward application of these designs will also provide an answer to the third question: Is this specific technique responsible for the observed behavior change? These points will be further elaborated in the final section of this chapter as will a general strategy for "untangling" complex intervention techniques to find the active change ingredient.

ABAB Design

The basic characteristics of the ABAB or reversal design are as follows: During the first A stage, a series of baseline observations are obtained on the target behavior; during the first B stage, the treatment or independent variable is manipulated while continual observations are taken on the target behavior; during the second A stage, or return to baseline, the treatment variable is removed, the procedures that were in effect during baseline are reinstituted, and observations continue. The last B stage is a return to the treatment procedure. (These four stages are depicted in Fig. 4-1.)

If the behavior is controlled by the experimental manipulations, it should rise and fall with each introduction and removal of the independent variable. (This is the pattern hoped for with acceleration programs. With deceleration programs, the opposite change direction would occur with each introduction and removal of the treatment variable.) Thus, in contrast to group designs where control is demonstrated by replicating *across subjects,* control in a reversal design is demonstrated by replicating *across conditions* for a single subject.

Illustration of ABAB design. We will illustrate the use of an ABAB design with an example in which the target behavior is the child's bed-making.

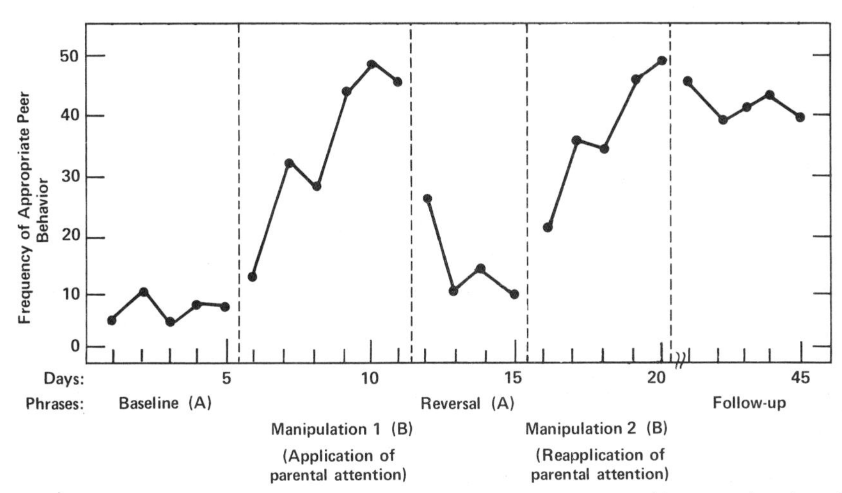

Fig. 4-1. Graph of appropriate interactions with peers (fictitious) using the reversal technique and a follow-up observation period. Figure taken from Hartmann (1969).

During the baseline period, daily observations are made of whether or not the child makes his bed. (If the child never makes his bed, we might decide to use a *retrospective baseline* rather than spending a week obtaining actual baseline, when that week could be better spent increasing bed-making. A retrospective baseline is one based on the verbal report of some responsible person such as the child's mother or teacher, rather than on formal observational procedures. Retrospective baselines should *only* be used when you can be certain that the behavior has either a zero rate or a 100 per cent rate of occurrence.) The number of days of baseline observations required is discussed in some detail in the chapter on data collection (Chapter 8).

During the B stage, the treatment manipulations (such as the use of instructions in conjunction with a point system for bed-making) are instituted. The duration of the treatment may vary from two or three days to two or three weeks or longer depending upon the success of the treatment, the stability of the target behavior, and the method used for graphing the data. (A suggested graphing technique for behaviors that can occur only once each day or for use when the baseline data are quite irregular, is to graph data by weeks rather than by days. If you decide to graph by weeks, you would want to carry out your treatment manipulation for at least one week, and probably for two or more weeks to get some idea of the weekly stability of the target behavior during treatment. Further information on graphing is included throughout the text and more specifically in Chapter 10 on data analysis.)

During the second A stage, or reversal period, the instructions and point system are removed and the conditions present during the baseline, (such as requests and nagging) are reestablished. Again, observations are continued throughout this stage until the behavior either reaches baseline level or has stabilized at some other level.

Finally, during the last stage, instructions and the point system are reinstated, and the desired rate of the target behavior recaptured.

The ABAB design is perhaps the most commonly used within-subject N=1 design in child behavior modification. The design has been used to demonstrate experimental control over behaviors as diverse as littering in a forest campground (Burgess, Clark, and Hendee, 1971), proper eating (O'Brien and Azrin, 1972), isolate behavior (Kirby and Toler, 1970), and racially integrated eating and play (Hauserman, Walen, and Behling, 1973). For additional examples of target behaviors and treatment techniques analyzed by means of the ABAB design and its variants, see recent issues of the *Journal of Applied Behavior Analysis.*

Advantages of the ABAB design. The basic advantage of a successful ABAB design is that it insures that changes in the child's behavior are due to the treatment manipulation rather than to some confounding variable (see section on threats to internal validity). For example, a rival interpretation to a treatment effect in a simple baseline-treatment or AB design is that the child changed because of some coincidental happening in his environment. However, each time we make a dramatic change in the rate of the target behavior, by introducing or removing the independent variable, the reasonableness of such an interpretation decreases. On occasion, we may want to expand the ABAB design by adding additional AB segments. Such expansion would be desirable when extraneous factors, which might conceivably be responsible for change in the child's behavior, occur simultaneously with our initial change from A to B and back to A. With the inclusion of enough AB segments, even the most skeptical become believers!

Another "rival" hypothesis in the simple AB design is that the repeated testing itself results in changes in the dependent variable. However, if the independent variable is introduced and removed a number of times with a subsequent rise and fall in the target behavior, the interpretation of repeated testing also loses credibility. The ABAB design, if conducted properly, also controls for the other previously described threats to internal validity, including maturation, instrument decay, and regression effects.

In addition to the technical advantages the ABAB design has for demonstrating control, it also may have therapeutic advantages. Baer et al. (1968, p.

94) suggest that repeated reversals may have a positive effect on the child subject by "contributing to the discrimination of relevant stimuli involved in the problem." Baer (1968) also suggests that the repeated reversal provides the behavior modifier with increased confidence in his ability to control behavior.

Limitations of the ABAB design. The most important limitations of the ABAB design are due to the *undesirability* of reversing some behaviors and the *"irreversibility"* of others.

Some behaviors such as fire-setting or self-destructiveness may be so serious that even a temporary resumption of these behaviors is totally unwarranted. Although you won't choose behaviors as serious as these to work with until you have moved from novice to journeyman status, the child's caretakers may be unwilling to approve of a temporary resumption of even a much milder problem behavior; be sure to discuss this matter with them early in your project. Even with minor problem behaviors and caretaker approval, one should be cautious in using this design repeatedly with a single child because inconsistency in child management techniques can be upsetting to the child. Although this typically may not be the case, you should be alert for emotional upset as a possible undesirable side effect.

Behaviors may be "irreversible" due to a number of causes:

1. Treatments may produce direct and irreversible behavior changes. For example, a surgical intervention may change the child's bodily structure so as either to prevent or to dramatically alter his capacity to emit certain target responses. Other more "psychological treatments may result in the acquisition of skill, such as reading or bicycle riding, which are not easily lost once acquired.

2. Treatments may continue to exert temporary effects even after they are withdrawn. Some drugs, for example, as well as certain intermittent schedules of reinforcement may continue to exert control over a behavior long after they have been withdrawn.

3. A response rate may be reversible, but not by reestablishing baseline conditions. For example, a child's ability to dress himself may be "self-reinforcing" and may not decrease even if the child is returned to a "baseline" environment in which the behavior is unreinforced by important caretakers.

4. Finally, it may not be possible to reinstitute external baseline *procedures.* For example, assume that during baseline conditions a nonverbal child worked with a teacher who refused to reinforce his grunts and other vocal approximations. Treatment might consist of a new teacher's using shaping and modeling procedures with the child. Thus, when his speech is well established and he is returned to his old teacher, his new verbal repertoire is generously reinforced by both his original teacher and his peers. Consequently, even though the treatment variables are removed, baseline procedures cannot

be reinstated, and the behavior will persist.

Because of the "irreversibility" of some behaviors, and the undesirability of reversing others, behavior modifiers have adopted alternative control procedures. Some of these procedures such as the DRO (Differential Reinforcement of Other behavior) and other rate-changing techniques described in Chapters 5 and 6 are employed when the behavior is reversible but not simply through reinstatement of baseline conditions (Baer and Wolf, 1970; Gelfand and Hartmann, 1968, p. 211). Still others, such as the multiple baseline procedures, are employed when the behavior either cannot or should not be reversed. The following section describes multiple baseline procedures, which fortunately, achieve control without temporarily decreasing the rate of desired behaviors.

Probe Questions for Part 2, Chapter 4

1. What functions are served by *each phase* of an ABAB design?

2. What is a retrospective baseline? When can a retrospective baseline be safely used?

3. Describe a situation in which more than two AB segments should be used in an experimental design.

4. What aspect of a reversal design might prove difficult for socializing agents to accept?

Behavioral Objectives for Part 3, Chapter 4

After reading Part 3 of this chapter, you should be able to:

1. State the defining characteristics of the multiple baseline design and the advantages and limitations of this design.

2. Select an appropriate design for your study.

Part 3. Within-Subject Designs: The Multiple Baseline and Alternative Designs

Multiple Baseline Designs

Multiple baseline designs typically involve keeping data on two or more behaviors that will be modified *sequentially* with the *same* treatment procedure. During the first step, then, baselines need to be obtained on each of the behaviors. During the next steps, one behavior at a time is manipulated, and data are continuously taken on the remaining behavior(s). Thus, if you were employing a positive reinforcement program to increase rates of three prosocial behaviors, you would consequate one of the target behaviors while continuing to take data on the other two. After a stable rate is achieved on the first consequated behavior, consequate behavior two while continuing to take baseline data on behavior three. Finally, consequate behavior three.

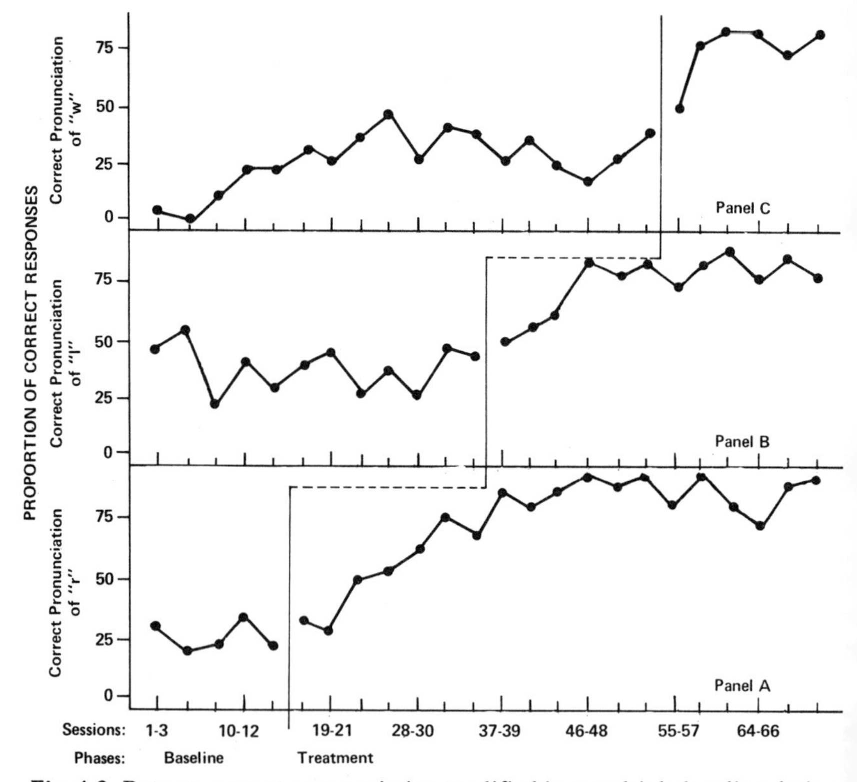

Fig. 4-2. Data on correct pronunciation modified in a multiple baseline design. Panel A shows data on "r" sound; Panel B shows data on "l" sound; Panel C shows data on "w" sound. (Data plotted are three day averages.)

Multiple baseline data, plotted for three-day averages on correct pronunciation of "r," "l," and "w" are shown in Fig. 4-2.
(*Note:* It is usually best to "piggyback" graphs when plotting the data from multiple baseline design studies – that is, each behavior is represented in a separate series of panels. The panels are aligned for easy comparison of rates of the different responses at the same moment in time. Putting more behaviors on a single graph often results in serious eyestrain for your readers. Compare, for example, Fig. 4-2 with Fig. 4-3.)

Figure 4-2 indicates how the baserate of each behavior is maintained until that behavior is itself manipulated. Control is then demonstrated by replicating a procedure *across a series of behaviors.* If each behavior remained at a fairly stable rate until it was administered the experimental treatment, you can safely assume that the treatment was responsible for the change in rate of that behavior.

Two other variants of the multiple baseline design are used in behavior modification studies. One version of this design requires the application of a treatment to one target response of a child under two or more stimulus conditions. Control is demonstrated by replicating a procedure *across a series of stimulus* conditions. The final version requires the application of a treatment to two or more subjects with the same target response and under the same environmental or stimulus conditions. Control is demonstrated by replicating a procedure *across a series of subjects.* These three types of multiple baseline designs are summarized in Table 4-1.

Table 4-1 Summary of Types of Multiple Baseline Designs

Control demonstrated by replicating across:	Number of Responses	Number of Settings	Number of Subjects
Responses	≥ 2	1	1
Settings	1	≥ 2	1
Subjects	1	1	≥ 2

Note: With each design, the same treatment procedure must be used consistently, whether across subjects, across settings, or across behaviors.

The three types of multiple baseline designs have only recently gained popularity in applied behavioral work with children, but their use is almost certain to increase. Surprisingly, most multiple baseline designs have employed multiple behaviors in a single setting, rather than a single behavior in multiple settings (see Jackson, 1973). Because the most commonly used form of this design requires the use of two or more behaviors that are likely to be similarly affected by a *single* treatment strategy, the range of behaviors for which this design is suitable is somewhat more restricted than is the case with the ABAB design. The behaviors over which control has been demonstrated in multiple baseline demonstrations include letter printing (Salzberg, Wheeler, Devar, and Hopkins, 1971), articulation errors (Bailey, Timbers, Phillips, and Wolf, 1971), imitative responding (Garcia, Baer, and Firestone, 1971), and fetishes (Marks and Gelder, 1967). The rationale for multiple baseline design and additional examples with children are described in recent papers by Hall, Cristler, Cranston, and Tucker (1970), Risley and Baer (1973), and Wolf and Risley (1971).

Illustration of a multiple baseline design. The target behavior we will use to illustrate the details of multiple baseline designs is aggressive play with siblings. This example demonstrates the second type of multiple baseline design in which a single response of a child is modified in three separate stimulus conditions: when the mother is the principal caretaker, when the father is the principal caretaker, and when a babysitter is the principal caretaker. The therapist would first obtain baserates on aggressive peer play under each of the three stimulus conditions or settings. It is important that interobserver reliability figures are obtained in each of the three settings – this is crucially important if the primary data gatherer is a different person in each of the three settings. This point will be amplified in the chapter on reliability. When the baselines become orderly (see Panel A in Fig. 4-3), the therapist would introduce the treatment into one of the three caretaker conditions. Which condition is treated first should be determined either randomly or, in this case, on the basis of whichever caretaker is least often responsible for the children. (See the section entitled "Limitations of the multiple baseline design" for an elaboration of this point.) In this example, we will assume a "traditional" household, and thus the child would probably be treated first in either the father or babysitter setting. Data would continue to be collected in all three settings. When the data have restabilized in the treated setting (see Panel B of Fig. 4-3), the therapist would introduce the treatment manipulation in the second condition, using a consistent criterion for selecting the second condition. If the choice of the first treatment setting was based on frequency of caretaker contact, this criterion would be used for selecting the second condition; if, instead, the random selection criterion had been used, it would continue to be used. When the rate had stabilized in this second condition (see Panel C of Fig. 4-3), the therapist would introduce the treatment in the remaining condition. Data would be collected until the rate in this condition had also stabilized (see Panel D of Fig. 4-3).

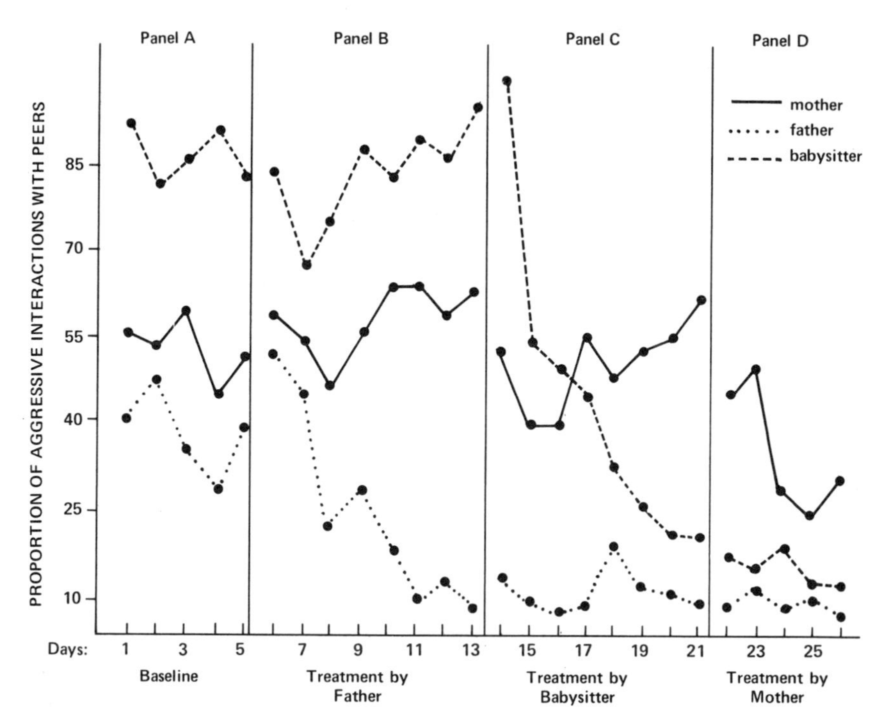

Fig. 4-3. Example of multiple baseline design showing proportions of aggressive peer interactions relative to total peer interactions in three stimulus conditions: with mother, with father, and with babysitter.

Advantages of the multiple baseline design. Whenever feasible in treatment demonstrations, it is safest to employ a multiple baseline procedure since it may be difficult or impossible to recapture baseline levels of performance in reversal (ABAB) designs (Risley, 1969; Sidman, 1960; and sad personal experience). If you have kept records on two or more target behaviors, and the rates of these behaviors were unaffected by the experimental manipulation, you can always resort to the multiple baseline model if your reversal procedure fails to produce the desired rate changes.

A second, and equally important advantage of the multiple baseline approach is that everyone is spared the painful process of reinstating some undesirable behavior, (for example, lying) solely in order to demonstrate the efficacy of the treatment procedure. Caretakers are usually only too glad to testify to the value of any intervention that has dealt successfully with a troublesome behavior, and they frequently don't appreciate the scientific and professional importance of an experimental demonstration. Caretakers are happier with a multiple baseline design. Not only is there no need to return to the old, unsatisfactory performance, but two or more desirable behaviors are instated for the price of one. A public relations dream come true.

Limitations of the multiple baseline design. One possible disadvantage of this design strategy is the additional time and effort it requires to collect multiple baseline data. The design also requires that each of the baseline rates should be relatively stable before initiation of the treatment program.

If you intend to use two or more behaviors, it may be difficult to find that many behaviors that can be treated with the same technique – a necessary prerequisite to using the multiple baseline approach. In general, behaviors of a single child that will be responsive to similar treatment strategies will be either topographically similar (e.g., saying "a," "o," and "u") or functionally similar (e.g., gaining attention by pulling on mother's apron, screaming at her, and kicking her in the shins).

It may also be difficult to find several behaviors that are independent, another requirement for a successful multiple baseline demonstration of control. By independence we mean that each behavior can be separately modified without changing the rate of the remaining unmodified behavior(s). Our concern with independence explains why we chose to manipulate aggressive peer play (see Fig. 4-3) initially in the least frequently occurring setting – with father. If, instead, we had first applied our treatment in the most frequently occurring setting (with mother), the treatment effect may have been more likely to *generalize* to the remaining untreated settings. If generalization had occurred, the opportunity to demonstrate experimental control would have been lost. For similar reasons, it would be unreasonable to use a multiple baseline design with a small child when the three target behaviors were tearing magazines, books, and papers. The child probably does not discriminate among the three behaviors, and so modifying book tearing would probably also affect magazine tearing. Independence as a requirement also implies that the behaviors cannot be developmental prerequisites for one another (Risley and Baer, 1973). For example, it would not be appropriate to choose standing, walking, and running as the three behaviors in a multiple baseline design for a one-year child. Because these behaviors occur in a developmental sequence, they would have to be "treated" in the order standing-walking-running. Even if they changed with the introduction of the treatment variable, experimental control would not be demonstrated; maturation would remain a threat to internal validity.

The checklist in Table 4-2 is for your use in determining which method of demonstrating control is most advisable for your project. After you have made a tentative decision based on the list, check with your instructor and get his approval. Whichever design you finally decide upon, remember the data gathering requirements of that design.

Table 4-2 Checklist for Determining Appropriate Method of Demonstrating Experimental Control

Necessary Requirements for ABAB Design:

_____Target behavior relatively innocuous (undesirable behavior can occur without dire results).

_____Parental approval obtained for worsening problem behavior after it has been brought under control.

_____Baseline conditions under your direct or indirect control and so can be reinstituted.

_____Control of the target behavior has not been gained by factors outside of the treatment context.

Unless you can meet each of the above requirements, do not use an ABAB design. Evaluate the possibility of a multiple baseline design.

Necessary Requirements for Multiple Baseline Design:

_____Time available to take baseline and continuous data on multiple responses.

_____Two or more responses for a single child, or a single response in either two or more settings or for two or more children, are available.

_____The rates of all target responses are likely to be independent.

Unless you have answered yes to each of these requirements, do not use a multiple baseline design. If neither the ABAB or multiple baseline technique is applicable to your problem, check with your instructor. You may have to change to a different target behavior.

OTHER EXPERIMENTAL DESIGNS

A number of writers discuss the limitations of both ABAB reversal and multiple baseline designs (e.g., Hartmann and Atkinson, 1973; Jones, 1974; Neale and Liebert, 1973; and O'Leary and Kent, 1973), such as (a) their stringent experimental control requirements, (b) the limited availability of appropriate statistical analysis techniques, (c) problems posed by carryover or order effects, and (d) sometimes questionable external validity. These problems have instigated the development of a number of other designs. Because these designs are used infrequently, we will describe each design only briefly and provide a reference to consult for further information.

Single subject randomization design. This design requires that each of two treatment conditions (or one treatment and one no-treatment condition) be repeatedly administered to a single subject in *random* order. This design can be safely employed only when the treatments are sufficiently spaced so that the response to a treatment is not affected by preceding treatments, and thus this approach has limited use in behavior modification studies. This design is described in some detail by Edgington (1969, pp. 135-140).

Multiple subject randomization design. Revusky (1967) describes a multiple subject design that shares some of the characteristics of both the multiple baseline and single subject randomization designs. This design requires baseline data for a single target behavior, such as remaining in seat, for each of at least four subjects. The treatment is then applied to each subject, but in a random order. Because this design requires a reasonably large number of subjects with identical target behaviors, it also is used infrequently in behavior modification work.

Quasi-experimental time series designs. A number of quasi-experimental time series designs using portions of either the reversal or multiple baseline design, such as a single AB component, are described by Gottman (1973), Campbell and Stanley (1963), and Glass, Willson, and Gottman (1972). While these designs have a role in exploratory work, they suffer from some of the major threats to internal validity previously described.

Stepwise criterion change design. Hartmann (1974 b) describes a variant of the multiple baseline design that requires stepwise changes in the rate of the target behavior corresponding to stepwise changes in the criteria for an adequate response. Control is then demonstrated by replicating a treatment program across a series of specified criteria. This design has not been used frequently enough for its utility to be fully known.

Probe Questions for Part 3, Chapter 4

1. Why might a multiple baseline design be preferred to a reversal design when peer aggression is the target behavior?

2. What are the requirements for a multiple baseline design?

3. How do the types of multiple baseline designs differ?

4. Why might a multiple baseline design foster good relations with parents and teachers?

Behavioral Objectives for Part 4, Chapter 4

After reading Part 4 of this chapter, you should be able to state how to establish simple cause-effect relationships between variables when complex intervention strategies are employed.

Part 4. Evaluating Complex Intervention Strategies

It may have occurred to you while reading the material on the ABAB and multiple baseline procedures that if the intervention procedures simply involved adding or omitting a *single* technique to what had been occurring during baseline, reliable observed changes in the target behavior could be attributed to that treatment technique. Thus, a specific cause-effect relationship between the target behavior and the technique could be asserted.

For example, assume that the behavior you had selected to increase was complying with requests. The child management technique used during baseline was a simple request from a caretaker whereas, during treatment, reinforcement for compliance was added to requests. If appropriately replicated, the increased rate of compliance during treatment could be attributed to the addition of the reinforcement contingency.

More frequently, however, treatment represents a change from one or more child management techniques (baseline procedure) to one or more different techniques during treatment. A caretaker may use belittling and spankings during baseline to control the rate of sibling aggression, and he may change during treatment to the use of a stimulus control procedure such as provision of rules plus positive reinforcement for cooperative interactions with siblings. Thus, one is left with a dilemma: Are changes in the target behavior due to (a) not doing what was done during baseline – in the previous example, not belittling and spanking, or (b) doing what was done during treatment – again referring back to our previous example, providing rules and reinforcing cooperative sibling interactions, or (c) both?

The general strategy for untangling complex changes in management procedures from baseline to treatment is to *manipulate one procedure at a time.* Before describing how one might apply this strategy to a specific problem, a word of warning is in order. If you plan to change a number of variables simultaneously, don't be upset if you have neither the time nor the inclination to engage in some fairly complicated untangling. The fact that your design stops short of determining a simple cause-effect relationship puts you in the therapy evaluation mainstream (Baer et al., 1968, p. 95). Certainly, do not choose a problem behavior simply because treatment will involve adding or deleting a single independent variable. A far better strategy is to maximize your probability of success. Perhaps the best way of doing that is to use a combination of treatment approaches – the blockbuster approach. By using this approach you will not only increase the probability of achieving success, but you will also expand your repertoire of treatment techniques at a time when you are both flexible and supervised.

Most of the information required to unravel complex intervention techniques is provided in this chapter and by the simple principle that sometime during your project one change will have to be made at a time. We will apply this information to one study to demonstrate how multiple treatment techniques might be individually evaluated. (This procedure is sometimes referred to as component analysis.)

For our example, consider a recent experiment by Cromer, Smith, Gelfand, Hartmann, and Page (1974), which attempted to demonstrate the effects of adult social consequences on children's willingness to aid another child. Our experience indicated that it would be necessary to include a "priming" technique, such as a verbal prompt, as well as adult approval to increase aiding (donating a token to a needy child) with children who failed to donate during baseline observations. Obviously, these children could not be

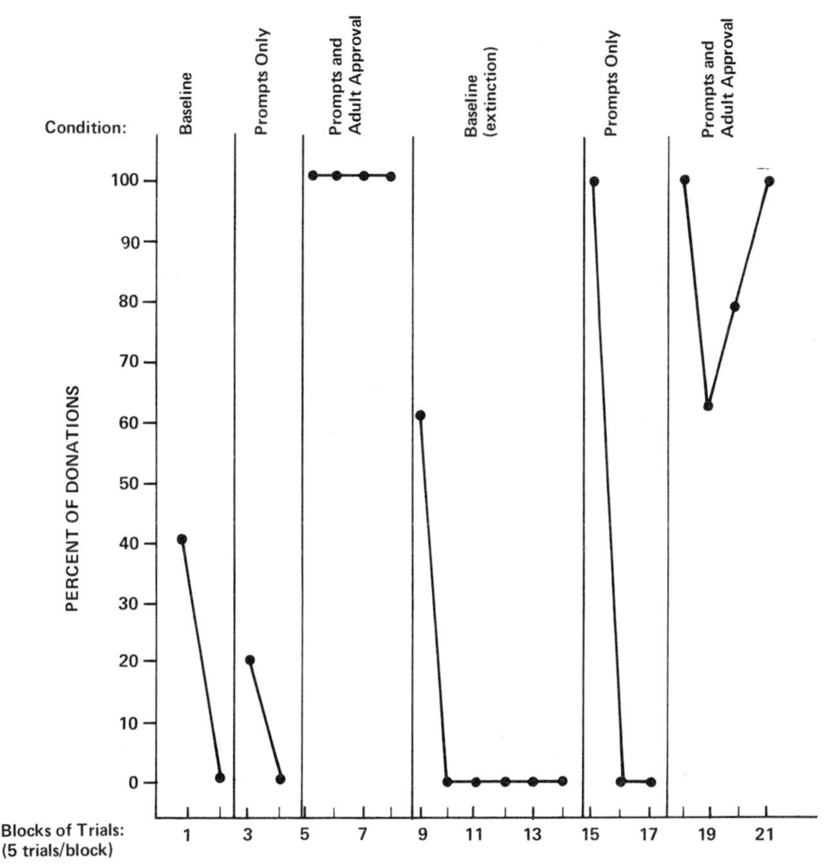

Fig. 4-4. An example of component analysis of the procedures used in. increasing children's aiding (donating). Data are taken from Cromer, Smith, Gelfand, Hartmann, and Page (1974).

reinforced for a response that never occurred. Because we were able to anticipate this problem, we initially designed the study in a manner to permit separate analyses of the effects of adult approval and of the effects of prompts (requests to donate). The sequence of conditions in the experimental design included (a) a short baseline, (b) "prompts only," (c) prompts plus contingent social approval, and finally (d) repetition of these three conditions. The data from a single child are shown in Fig. 4-4. While it still might be argued that it was repeated prompts and not the contingent social approval that maintained help-giving at a high rate, other investigators' results (e.g., Hopkins, 1968), as well as data from other subjects who had failed to respond despite repeated prompts, suggested that this interpretation was unlikely.

The ease with which baseline rates were recaptured in this example is a distinct advantage for purposes of demonstrating control. It is a disadvantage in another sense: We hope that when a behavior is modified by some contrived arrangement of contingencies, the contrived contingencies can be removed quickly and the behavior will continue because it is now either self-sustaining or is maintained by natural external consequences. Baer and Wolf (1967) use the term "behavioral trap" to refer to an environment in which naturally occurring consequences will take over and maintain newly acquired responses. When natural contingencies do not support newly acquired behaviors, additional treatment, perhaps in the form of extensive environmental engineering, would have to continue in order for durable change to occur (see Chapters 5 and 9 for details). The apparent contradictions between the clinician's hope that natural contingencies gain control of the target behavior and the researcher's hope that he will be able to demonstrate control has been discussed in a recent paper by Hartmann and Atkinson (1973).

As can be seen from this example, component analysis involves no new design principles. The untangling strategy is a simple one: isolate the components in the treatment package to determine which one or more is responsible for the change. Examples of component analyses in applied behavior modification are given in Baer and Wolf (1970), in Risley and Wolf (1973), and in occasional articles in the *Journal of Applied Behavior Analysis.* Useful but more general reviews of methodological issues in behavior therapy research can be found in McNamara and MacDonough (1972) and Paul (1969).

Probe Questions for Part 4, Chapter 4

1. What are the advantages and disadvantages of the single-variable intervention approach and the "blockbuster" approach?

2. What is a component analysis?

3. The easy reversal of a behavior in an ABAB design can be a boon to the researcher and a threat to the clinician. Explain this statement.

4. Design a component analysis to assess independently the effects of verbal instructions, physical prompts, and a positive reinforcement contingency, all of which in combination have been successfully used to increase the rate of some prosocial behavior.

Behavioral Objectives for Part 1, Chapter 5

When you have read Part 1 of this chapter, you should be able to:

1. Choose the behavior modification agent most appropriate for the situation, and provide a rationale for your choice of agent.

2. Become acquainted with the child so that he will respond well to the treatment program.

3. Arrange a favorable learning environment.

CHAPTER 5

Increasing Deficit Behavior

Part 1. General Considerations in Initiating a Treatment Program

CHOICE OF MODIFICATION AGENT

It is sometimes difficult to decide which person should best carry out a modification program with a child. The child's ordinary caretakers (such as his parents and his teacher) have some obvious advantages as modification agents. First of all, they are and have been the child's instructors in numerous academic and social skills. Thus, they frequently have a valuable store of experience in the types of tactics that are most effective with this particular child. They already have an established relationship with him, in most cases a positive one. Thus, their attention is a generalized conditioned reinforcer, which can be made contingent upon the desired behavior.

Furthermore, the caretakers are with the child for large portions of nearly every day, so that they can easily administer scores of learning trials to him in relatively short periods of time. Long after the student therapist has terminated his relationship with the child, the caretakers can continue the treatment program. As we shall point out in Chapter 9, there are also fewer problems in generalization of treatment effects when the adult care agents administer the training. Therefore, in terms of relationship variables, availability, convenience, generalization, and program duration, parents and teachers are frequently the modification agents of choice.*

*Helpful reviews of the use of parents and teachers as behavior change agents have been written by Berkowitz and Graziano (1972), Johnson and Katz (1973), and by O'Dell (1974). While they are primarily research oriented, these reviews can acquaint you with some of the techniques that have been found effective in the training and supervision of parents acting as therapists.

But what does the student therapist have to offer? A knowledge of basic behavior principles upon which to base an effective treatment strategy, an awareness of the importance of consistency of procedures and of accurate and faithful observation and data collection, and no previous history of having failed to control the problem behavior. If the caretakers and the child are at loggerheads over the target behavior, the more objective, less emotional student therapist can treat the situation calmly and allow the others to withdraw from combat with honor.

In addition, we have not yet begun to examine the disadvantages of caretakers as therapists. Their attitudes about proper child behavior can prevent them from acting therapeutically. Some of them consider it undesirable if not downright sinful to materially reward or even to praise the child for "things he should already be doing anyway." This is clearly a misconception of the principles governing children's behavior (Gelfand, 1969, pp. 175-176), an opinion that is often easier to change through a demonstration of an improvement in the child's behavior than through scientific or logical arguments. Although they may not be resistant to your doing so, the caretakers may not themselves choose knowingly to reinforce the child for good behavior, at least not initially. If this is the case, your program might stand little chance of implementation at the hands of the child care agents.

Or, suppose the caretakers agree with the philosophy of your program, does this presuppose their success as therapists? Not unless they can carry out the procedures accurately and reliably. It is nearly a sure bet that they cannot do so without considerable training and supervision from you. The process is particularly difficult if the caretaker is already very busy. Even with the best will in the world, a classroom teacher with 40 youngsters on her hands may find it difficult to initiate a behavior modification program with one particular child. There are simply too many competing demands on her time.

Also remember that in instructing caretakers, you will be attempting to shape complex new childrearing behaviors without powerful reinforcers at your command. Your unsubstantiated promise that the procedures you recommend will improve the situation may not suffice if the procedures in question prove distasteful, time consuming, and dull, which is sometimes the case. Remember that behavior principles apply in work with parents and teachers as well as with children. If you have no previously established relationships with the child's caretakers, and can offer them no appealing incentive to cooperate, you may have to spend more time than is desirable in pleading and cajoling to see that they carry out the program. If you are too demanding, they may simply withdraw their cooperation; if you are too ready to compromise, the diluted modification program may fail.

Then there are some other considerable advantages in conducting the treatment program yourself. You will probably gain experience in basic behavior modification skills, such as data collecting and shaping. You will learn the many informal skills involved in working directly with children. You will be able to change the program more quickly and easily should it prove ineffective, and you will be completely aware of the teaching techniques used – that is, you will not have to rely on the sometimes inaccurate reports of the caretakers. From the educational standpoint, you have much to gain from acting as the modification agent yourself.

In summary, then, our advice is that you act as the primary therapist working directly with the child. This is particularly applicable to your first attempts at behavior modification. Those with prior experience can profitably direct caretakers and others in the use of behavior modification techniques. Only in cases in which you have a prior and continuing relationship with the caretakers (e.g., when you are a colleague, preferably a supervisor), is it advisable to attempt to have your *first* modification program carried out by others.

SET UP A FAVORABLE LEARNING SITUATION

You can make life much easier for yourself and the learning task easier for the child by setting up a favorable environment for learning. In simplest terms, this means that the setting should be as pleasant as possible with few or no extraneous stimuli competing for the child's attention.

Get Acquainted with the Child

Ordinarily, you cannot expect to begin your acquaintance with your child-client with the first learning trial of your therapeutic program. You must first establish yourself as a friendly, rewarding person and the training situation as a nonthreatening one. Otherwise, the child may be so intimidated and frightened by the prospect of facing a strange adult in unfamiliar circumstances that he may fail to attend to the training stimuli you are attempting to present. Even investigators who work with animals must first accustom their subjects to handling, to the experimental chamber, and to the operation of the food and water dispenser. With children, the acquaintance process is perhaps even more important to the success of the program, since they and their caretakers are free to withdraw their involvement at any time.

In order to appear less intimidating to the child, you should approach him in his customary environment. After introducing yourself and chatting with him, you might attempt to engage him in some entertaining activity. Do something that you will enjoy as well. Perhaps you could introduce some interesting project such as building a model airplane or making a clay sculpture or a collage. If you sing or play a musical instrument, you could perform children's songs, folk songs, or popular songs with him. If you can do folk dances or modern dance, you might engage him in these activities. Games and sports such as playing catch, bowling, shooting baskets, or practicing gymnastics are also good bets. These activities are not only relaxing and fun for the youngster but also might add to your status with him if you demonstrate some skill at them. If he really enjoys one of these activities, you may be able to use it later contingently as a reinforcing event for him.

If you will be using candy or toys in your treatment procedure, give him some now. This act will both help you determine their reinforcing value and will associate your presence with the availability of reinforcing events. You will become discriminative for approach rather than avoidance on the child's part. Remember also that if you are working with a partner both of you must become acquainted with the child since you will both act as therapists.

If you are unfamiliar with the ways of children and don't know how best to approach them, observe the teachers and others who have a good relationship with the child. How do they interact with him when they want him to enjoy himself? They might also be willing to offer you some good suggestions. For possible children's games and play activities you might use, browse through copies of the journal *Childhood Education* or consult any one of a number of available books on the topic (e.g., American Association for Health, Physical Education, and Recreation, 1964; Arnold, 1968; Association for Childhood Education International, 1964; Buist and Schulman, 1969; Donnelly and Mitchell, 1958; Hartley and Goldenson, 1963; Kraus, 1957; Latchaw, 1970). The Arnold book is widely available in a paperback edition. When you and the child become fairly comfortable with each other, it is time for your therapeutic program to begin.

Explain the Program to the Child

We recommend as full a disclosure to the child as is possible regarding the purposes and procedures of your program. If your aim is to help reduce the number of commands and threats a child issues in order to make him a more attractive companion to classmates, tell him so. Make every attempt, of course, to preserve his dignity in the process so that he does not feel unduly threatened or become defensive. Tell him that it is like a music lesson or a school lesson, but that in this instance he is learning how to help other people and himself get along well. Because such explanations require great tact and social skill, many therapists avoid offering the child any reasons for their presence or their requests. This practice makes the whole process appear mysterious and arbitrary to the child. We feel that it is desirable to explain as much about the program as is consistent with the child's age and ability to understand and with the goals of the treatment intervention.

A Partner Aids in Data Collection

As was pointed out in Chapter 1, a partner who can assist you in your data collection is a significant asset during the first several treatment sessions. It is very difficult to keep an eye on the child, find the stimulus materials, control the reinforcers, and record data at the same time, particularly when you are a novice at all of these activities. A data-recording partner can significantly decrease your burden during these early sessions and allow you to concentrate on the child and the program. The situation you face is somewhat analogous to learning to juggle three oranges; the feat can be learned best by starting with one orange, then two, and finally working up to the complex task of dealing with three at once. So it is with all the materials you must manage simultaneously when conducting your program and recording data. You can make your work easier by not overloading yourself at first.

A partner also serves a useful function as a friendly critic. Being unimpeded by the demands of carrying out the program while you are acting as therapist, he can also note the quality of your general interactions with the child. He can let you know whether or not you appear friendly to the child, whether your rate of presentation of learning trials is appropriate, whether you are consistent in the use of reinforcement criteria, and whether you abide by the written program script (to be described later).

In case unforeseen difficulties arise, and they nearly always do, you can consult with each other concerning the best way to deal with them. Since both of you will have witnessed the problem, you will be better able to develop a successful plan for its resolution.

It is also easier to standardize your training procedures if both you and your partner can be present at the initial sessions. Otherwise you might each devise separate and different procedures, which could complicate and hinder your modification efforts. In order to relieve the burden on the beginning behavior modifier and to standardize procedures, it is best for both partners in the therapist pair to attend the initial treatment sessions.

Location for Individual Sessions

If you will be engaging in one-to-one tutoring with the child, find a location that will maximize his attending to the learning task. The location you select should be convenient, quiet, and well-illuminated. It should be private so that intruders do not distract you or the child. And the child should be positioned so that he can neither hear nor see other interesting activities he might prefer. This means that if there is a window allowing a view of a playground, the child should be seated with his back to the view. Perhaps the shades should be drawn before the child enters the room so that he has no opportunity to sample the appealing vista outside.

Apparatus preparation. If possible, have the room in order before you escort the child in to begin each treatment session. Have your materials set out on the table before the child arrives. Since you will be keeping data on his performance, have a clipboard with the prepared data sheet and a pencil ready, or have some alternative data collection apparatus set up for use immediately upon the child's entrance. This means that you can devote your full attention to the child and not be fumbling around looking for a pencil while he waits and perhaps gets into mischief.

Have your reinforcers ready for dispensing and in sufficient quantity so that you do not run out of them during the session. Have them located so that they are out of the child's reach and his line of vision. Otherwise, he may attend to the reinforcers rather than to you and the task at hand. And you certainly do not want to get into a wrestling match with him over possession of the reinforcers.

Finally, remember to have the stimulus materials ready in the order in which you wish to present them. If you are using picture cards in a naming task, for example, have the cards arranged in the proper order prior to the session. Fumbling is aversive for both you and the child. A good general policy is to avoid much moving of furniture or the use of complex or delicate equipment that you must maintain and guard against damage.

Conducting classroom or home projects. You will have somewhat less control over the situation if the modification program is to be conducted during the child's normal home or school activities rather than in a specially prepared tutoring setting. Nevertheless, the same principles hold. Try to insure that no one else is attempting a competing behavior control procedure at the same time. Your reinforcement program is hampered if the child's father threatens him with a spanking if he does not start cooperating with his little brother, or if the mother nags the child constantly about not doing his homework. Similarly, if a teacher continues an ineffectual punishment tactic with the child while you are trying to shape his attending to academic materials, your program will suffer. You must make sure that everyone has agreed that your program, and only your program, will be put into effect to deal with this particular target behavior. This will frequently require as much tact and persuasiveness as you can exert.

Stimulus control. It is frequently quite difficult to identify all of the stimulus events that are serving as SD's for a particular child behavior. For example, in the case of study behavior, the SD's involved may include the color, texture, size, and weight of the textbooks, the presence of the teacher and classmates, and the physical characteristics of the classroom. Unfortunately, all of these stimuli could also serve as SD's for gazing off into space or throwing spitwads. In circumstances in which you suspect that a whole variety of stimuli are serving as SD's for a child's undesirable behavior, you might want to help promote behavior change by fitting your tutoring area and your teaching materials with stimulus characteristics widely at variance with the child's usual surroundings. You might provide a colorful flowered cover for a dull, grey, exercise book; the child might be given colored rather than ordinary lead pencils to write with, and he might do his studying in a special room or study area rather than at his accustomed desk. It is also advisable, at least initially, to conduct the treatment session in the same location and at the same time each day in order to establish strong stimulus control over the youngster's behavior. Then, gradually, the stimuli present in his ordinary environment can be faded into his surroundings so that eventually he is using his everyday study materials and is situated in his old location.

Timing. The time of day you select for your treatment sessions can also have a considerable bearing on your success. Select a time when the child is neither fatigued nor eager to go to recess or return home from school. If your program involves the use of food reinforcers, it is important to conduct sessions at times when the child is at least moderately hungry, certainly not immediately after a meal time.

Timing considerations will affect your relationship with caretakers also. Try to minimize your intrusion on their schedules. This means that you should not hold training sessions in the home during the child's (or the parents') favorite television program, nor make the family delay dinner so that they are exposed to appetizing cooking odors while you are trying to eliminate sulkiness and quarreling among siblings. Insofar as possible, schedule around competing attractive activities and eliminate competing modification efforts wherever your program takes place.

Fatigue or hunger may affect your performance as well. If possible, select a session time at which you will not be overly pressed for time and will be at your best. Realistically, at certain times of the academic year, students never feel unpressured or carefree. Therefore, if this last advice is laughable in your current situation, turn the page without a qualm.

Probe Questions for Part 1, Chapter 5

1. Suppose you wished to teach a young child to eat with a spoon rather than with his fingers. How would you set up an optimal learning environment for him?

2. Describe the conditions under which each of the following persons would be the best choice of modification agents: a parent, a teacher, a student therapist.

3. Why is it a good idea to conduct a modification project with a partner rather than to work alone?

4. Drawing upon your own recreational skills and interests, plan a set of activities that would help you become a possible source of reinforcement for (a) a four-year-old boy, (b) a ten-year-old girl, (c) the child with whom you are considering working.

Behavioral Objectives for Part 2, Chapter 5

Study of Part 2 of this chapter should enable you to:

1. Define and identify reinforcing events.

2. State the characteristics of a reinforcer useful in a treatment program.

3. Prevent a child-client from becoming quickly satiated with a reinforcer used in treatment.

4. Establish conditioned reinforcing properties for selected stimuli, e.g., tokens or points.

5. Answer the most commonly voiced objections to the use of tangible reinforcers with children.

Part 2. Identifying or Establishing Reinforcing Events

Since the treatment of most behavioral deficits involves the administration of reinforcing events, we will describe in some detail the process of reinforcer selection and the establishment and use of conditioned and generalized reinforcers. In succeeding sections we will present material on the shaping, modeling, and contingency contracting techniques involved in devising and implementing a treatment program for teaching a child new behavioral skills.

REINFORCING EVENTS

People who are unfamiliar with behavior modification often assume that the task of selecting a reinforcer is an easy one. "Don't you just give the child a candy or say 'Good?' " they ask. Unfortunately, the process is rarely that simple. Since reinforcing events are, by definition, identified behaviorally rather than rationally, one cannot conclusively select a reinforcer for a particular child in advance of observation. A reinforcer is any stimulus event that is effective in producing an increase in the recurrence of a preceding behavior. Therefore, only by observation of an individual's response rates can we determine the reinforcing or nonreinforcing characteristics of a given stimulus. Further, even for a particular child, different stimulus events may serve as reinforcers at different times. The child's relative states of satiation and deprivation play important roles in determining the momentary strength of a potential reinforcing event. Thus, the same candy a child works for eagerly at 3 p.m. he may view with disdain at 7 p.m. just after he has finished a large dinner. The factors of individual preference plus the influence of setting events sometimes make reinforcer identification a difficult task.

Premack's Principle

Acquaintance with Premack's Differential Probability Principle (Premack, 1959) is a great help in the search for reinforcers. Simply stated, this principle holds that for any two behaviors emitted by an organism, the lower rate behavior can be made more probable by making contingent upon its occurrence the opportunity to engage in the higher rate behavior. Thus, if a child plays baseball readily (high-rate behavior) but rarely practices the piano (low-rate behavior), you can increase his music practice by making the opportunity to play baseball contingent upon piano practice. As a behavior analyst, then, your role is to discover the child's naturally occurring high-rate behaviors, whatever they might be (Homme and Tosti, 1965).

How to Identify Reinforcers

Observation. If the child's target behavior is a high-rate, undesirable one, you might use your behavior observations to identify the reinforcers maintaining it. Then you might alter the situation so that these reinforcers are instead made contingent upon some lower rate desirable behavior. In other words, your behavior observations can yield information on stimulus events serving as reinforcers for your child-client. If his disruptive behavior seems to be maintained by teacher attention, you might wish to select teacher attention as the reinforcer to be used in your modification program.

You might also wish to make a special observation of the child's free play to identify his favorite activities. Provide a selection of toys, games, and foods. Then note how much time he spends at each activity. Does he smile, exclaim that he likes it, ignore opportunities to engage in other behaviors, try to keep it to himself and guard it closely, or, perhaps, offer to share it as a special favor? If he displays one or more of these behaviors, the activity in question might be used as a reinforcing event.

Interviews. Interviews with the caretakers and with the child himself are helpful in providing clues regarding usable reinforcers. Appendix B provides a checklist that caretakers or children could be asked to complete to indicate the child's preferences. Cautela and Kostenbaum (1967) have provided a similar checklist for use with adolescents and adults. Madsen and Madsen (1972) have also recently offered extensive lists of suggested approval and disapproval responses to be used in consequating child behavior.

If you wish to conduct a brief interview, you might ask the following questions regarding the child client:

What are (child's name)'s favorite foods or snacks?
What are his favorite candies?
What are his favorite kinds of drinks?
What games and sports does he enjoy playing? Enjoy watching?
What toys does he prefer? Which ones would he like to buy if he could?
Which books, magazines, or comics does he like?
Who are his favorite friends among children? Among adults?
What nearby points of interest does he like to visit? (for example, parks, zoos, lakes and streams, amusement parks)
Does he like to play with or care for pets? Which ones?
Does he have any favorite television programs? Does he like movies?
What are his hobbies?

Characteristics of a Useful Reinforcer

By this time you will probably have discovered a number of different stimulus events that you could use as reinforcers. But some are more useful than others. The reinforcers most easily utilized in treatment programs possess the following characteristics:

1. *Reinforcer is resistant to satiation.* Reinforcer satiation presents one of the greatest problems associated with the use of reinforcers in modification programs. Whether they take place in the classroom, the family, or in a private setting, programs are usually devised so that the child is presented with many learning trials in each treatment session. If he rapidly becomes satiated with the proferred reinforcing stimulus, the potential number of learning trials is significantly decreased as is the rate of his behavior change. Therefore, it is essential to combat satiation effects. There are several ways to do this.

First, rather than using just one type of reinforcing stimulus, offer some variety. For example, you might want to use some combination of candy, nuts, water, juice, gold stars, toys, attention, and smiles as reinforcers. The variety helps to counteract both momentary satiation and longer term preference changes. One useful method for presenting a selection of potential reinforcers is the Reinforcing Event Menu (Addison and Homme, 1966). If you are working with a young child, you can present him with a cardboard card similar to a restaurant menu and featuring pictures of the various stimulus events you are offering as reinforcers. He makes his choice and you contract with him concerning exactly how much and what type of work he must complete to earn that reward. In work with older children, you can present the menu in written rather than in pictorial form, or you can describe it orally.

Second, you can keep your training sessions relatively brief, e.g., ten to 15 minutes with preschool children and no longer than 30 minutes with older children. It is usually more effective in achieving rapid progress to hold daily 10-minute training sessions than a weekly one-hour training session. The former training schedule's superiority is probably due to the daily practice plus the accompanying minimal satiation effects. Brief and frequent sessions also allow you to change you tactics more readily if you discover that your procedures require changes.

A third, and highly effective method for preventing satiation involves the use of conditioned generalized reinforcers such as tokens, points, money, or verbal approval. Since conditioned and generalized reinforcers are so frequently used in modification programs, they will be discussed more fully in a following section. Readers interested in information on additional methods for avoiding reinforcer satiation are referred to Bijou and Baer (1966).

2. *Reinforcer can be adminstered in small units.* Reinforcer administration should occur frequently and in small units. It is usually a much better practice to reinforce the child frequently with small sips of soft drink, for example, than to offer him a giant Coke but only at long intervals. Some therapists have found a plastic squirt dispenser a handy instrument for dispensing juice or soft drink. The spout of the squirt dispenser is placed very close to or inside the child's mouth, and a small amount of juice is injected. Offering a larger amount of the reinforcer, but infrequently and for large units of work, can result in ratio strain and consequent disruption or collapse of performance. So chop your M&M candies into small pieces, dispense your soft drinks by the squirt or the eye-dropper-full, keep the play opportunities brief, or the value of each token low, and your program will prosper as long as the child is not being underpaid for his efforts.

3. *Reinforcer can be administered immediately after occurrence of desired behavior.* You are usually in bad straits if you are using as a back-up reinforcer the opportunity to view a TV program that appears only once a week or some other such infrequent reinforcement opportunity. Such a long time intervenes between the child's desirable performance and the reinforcing event that you cannot tell which of the child's responses are being effectively reinforced. Suppose he had just hit his little brother immediately prior to the broadcast of the TV show. In that event, if he gets to see the show, he might be reinforced for hitting his brother. If he does not get to see the show because of his misbehavior, you have broken your agreement with him and have failed to reinforce his previous desirable performance. What to do? Reinforce as quickly as possible after the desirable performance. This is particularly important early in the training program. Later, the duration of the interval between performance and reinforcement can gradually be increased somewhat. When you do use a delay, be sure to tell the child what he is being reinforced for. In at least some instances, you can remind the child of what he has done, and then reinforce him for his past performance.

4. *Reinforcer administration is exclusively under the treatment agent's control.* Suppose that you as the treatment agent are using candy-coated bubble gum as a reinforcer. Now suppose that the child's Aunt Martha has given him a toy bubble gum dispenser for his birthday so that he has free access to all the gum he wants. What do you think this will do to your program? It is frequently advisable to ask the child's parents to limit his access to the reinforcing stimulus for the duration of the program or at least to inform you if something like the Aunt Martha episode does occur. This is not to imply that you should attempt to deny the child his favorite activities for the duration of your project. If possible, select reinforcing stimuli that are over and above those that he can expect on an everyday basis. Otherwise, the

child may correctly perceive you as denying him his customary pleasures – a situation not calculated to elicit his full cooperation.

During the training sessions themselves, you must make sure that you, not the child, control the administration of the reinforcers, both as regards their timing and quantity. Hold on to the candy bowl; do not put it on the table beside the child and expect him to refrain from helping himself. At the inception of the modification program, you must establish that you, and you alone, control the flow of goodies, which is dependent upon his correct response.

5. *Reinforcer is compatible with treatment program.* Do not use a reinforcer that will compete with the very behavior you are intending to instate. For example, do not use peanut butter as a reinforcer in a speech articulation training program; do not use candy as a reinforcer in a weight control program, or aggressive play activities to reinforce cooperative behavior in a hyperaggressive child.

6. *Reinforcer is practical.* Choose reinforcers that are not too costly, that have no undesirable side effects, that are easily transported, and that are readily available in large supply.

Conditioned Reinforcers

Conditioned reinforcers often meet the previously suggested criteria of being resistant to satiation and dispensible in small units immediately following the desired performance. A conditioned reinforcer acquires its reinforcing properties through being paired with another reinforcing event, so many different stimuli can become conditioned reinforcers. For example, a particular sound, a facial expression, a pat on the back, or a plastic poker chip might each precede and signal the availability of some reinforcer. The latter is frequently termed a back-up reinforcer. If conditioned reinforcers are associated with a variety of other types of reinforcers, they become *generalized* conditioned reinforcers. Praise, tokens, or points typically precede or can be exchanged for many types of back-up reinforcers. Consequently, these generalized reinforcers maintain their reinforcing properties over various deprivation types and levels. This characteristic is a distinct advantage in a therapy program as the following example illustrates. If you have paired a simple, conditioned reinforcer (points earned) only with the availability of candy, and the child has already consumed many candies, he probably won't work to acquire the conditioned reinforcer. If instead you have paired the conditioned reinforcer, points, with the availability of a number of other reinforcers (food, special clothing, entertainment, social recognition), his momentary satiation on candy would not preclude his working to earn the generalized conditioned reinforcer.

Generalized reinforcers also: (a) serve as a means for bridging some delay between a performance and back-up reinforcement, (b) can be administered flexibly and continuously throughout the day, and (c) may even take on greater incentive value than would a single primary reinforcer because of their association with a number of different back-up reinforcers. (See Kazdin and Bootzin [1972] for a more detailed discussion of the advantages associated with use of generalized conditioned reinforcers.)

Because of these many desirable qualities, generalized reinforcers are frequently used in treatment programs. Fortunately, for many children the job of establishing conditioned reinforcers has already been accomplished. Their families, friends, and teachers have already made praise, smiles, and other forms of attention generalized conditioned reinforcers. Since praise can often be delivered promptly and flexibly without disruption of on-going activities, it is frequently employed in shaping procedures with children. This does not mean, however, that you can assume that you can use it effectively with a child who is a stranger to you. You must first become socially acquainted with the child, and frequently you must also offer him attractive reinforcers paired with your praise before you can proceed to use praise alone effectively in a training venture. Omitting this important first step may result in your praise to the child acting as a neutral or even aversive stimulus. This would, of course, negate your treatment efforts.

Implementation. Let us suppose that you have discovered that your praise does not function as a reinforcer for your child-client, and that you wish to establish some stimulus such as a plastic poker chip as a conditioned reinforcer. First, you establish the chip as valuable by giving the child a chip and immediately allowing him to exchange it for a play privilege, a treat, or some other reinforcer. You may do this several times, each time telling him, "You can play with the hamster a while [or whatever reinforcing event is being used] if you have a chip." Then you can tell him how to earn one. You might say, "Now every time you can tell me the name of the animal in the picture, you will get one chip." Next give him one trial to earn a token and then allow him to exchange his token for the back-up reinforcer. Repeat this process until the token itself functions as a reinforcer. In working with a more skilled (or older) child, you may just be able to instruct him that he will have an opportunity to turn in his tokens for the back-up reinforcers in a little while or after the training session. The exact instructions you use will depend upon the child's vocabulary and his social skills.

Since the object in using a token reinforcer is to initiate the desired performance, not to keep the child on a token program permanently, you must immediately begin establishing praise as an additional conditioned reinforcer. The very first time and each time, that you present the child with a token reinforcer, you must precede it with a big smile and some positive comment about how smart the child is, how well he is doing, or some other pleasant remark. So you will say, "Right on, Willie! That's an elephant. Smart boy!" and you will hand him his token or make a tally mark on his paper. Praise precedes the other conditioned reinforcer, and so acquires conditioned reinforcing properties itself. At first, you may want to exaggerate your praise and smiling so that the child will be more likely to attend to them. Eventually, you will aim to reduce and finally eliminate the use of the token reinforcer, and maintain the improved behavior on occasional praise alone, a naturally occurring contingency.

The elimination of the artificial reinforcement procedure proceeds by gradual stages. For continuous performances, such as the child's remaining seated during classroom instruction, the child might initially be reinforced with tokens on the average of once each minute for staying seated. This schedule of reinforcement is referred to as a variable interval one minute or VI 1' schedule. The range of time intervals might vary between a minimum of 15 sec., and a maximum of 85 sec. (see, for example, Christy, 1973). The average duration of this schedule could be progressively increased in increments not readily detected by the child, until at last he receives no token reinforcement. A similar procedure of thinning reinforcement schedules can be used with training tasks involving discrete trials such as occur in many language instruction programs. Initially the tokens are administered for each correct response; this is, on a continuous reinforcement (CRF) schedule. When the child is responding correctly on 80 percent or more of the training trials for two or three consecutive days, reinforcement can be administered for every other correct response. An intermittent reinforcement schedule in which every n^{th} correct response is reinforced is called a fixed ratio (FR) schedule. Reinforcing every second correct response produces a FR2 schedule. When the intermittent schedule is first used, there may be a decrement in the child's performance. If necessary, stable correct responding should be re-established; then the therapist should introduce greater variability and intermittency by reinforcing the child on the average of every third or every fourth correct response – a variable ratio (VR) 3 or 4 schedule. Increasing intermittency can be introduced progressively until tokens are no longer needed to maintain the target behavior.

It is important to bring the child to the point at which his appropriate behavior is maintained on a schedule and with a type of reinforcement similar to that occurring in his usual classroom or home environment. Otherwise, his newly established performance might collapse as he encounters a naturalistic situation greatly at variance with that of the therapeutic program. Further details on procedures for fading from the artificial treatment environment to the child's natural environment are presented in Chapter 9.

Sometimes, of course, the customary environment does not provide sufficient reinforcement to maintain the child's desirable behavior regardless of how carefully the therapeutic program is phased out. In the total absence of natural reinforcement contingencies, it may be necessary to attempt to train caretakers or peers in how and when to administer reinforcement. While it involves no new principles, this latter task is complex and difficult, and we do not recommend it for novice therapists. Should you discover that the natural environment lacks any reinforcement for your client's prosocial behavior, consult with your instructor on how best to proceed.

The matter of reinforcer prices charged the child and his rates of pay are complex ones and call for the skills of a practicing economist. You must pay the child enough to keep him working diligently, but not overpay him so that he need not work long in order to earn his reinforcers. Walker and Buckley (1974) suggest some helpful guidelines for setting initial wages and prices in a classroom token reinforcement system. These writers suggest an average hourly wage for acceptable work of 5 cents for elementary school children, 10 cents for junior high school students, and 15 cents for those in high school. These rates don't appear overgenerous, but apparently are sufficiently attractive to induce the children to work for them. Walker and Buckley initially charge their child-clients the actual cost of purchased items such as games, toys, or edible treats. Recreational activities are priced at between 5 and 15 minutes of activity time in exchange for the amount the child would earn in one hour. The suggested initial ratio of tokens to cents is five tokens for each cent, so a 5 cent item would require the child to earn 25 tokens, a 10 cent item, 50 tokens, and so forth. This exchange rate allows the therapist to award tokens frequently at the inception of the program. The child may also be allowed to exchange his tokens for back-up reinforcers several times a day at first, then gradually be introduced to a more intermittent exchange schedule. This increasing delay must be imposed quite gradually, and if it seems to be momentarily disrupting the child's performance (i.e., if he performs erratically or stops performing altogether), you must resume the more frequent exchanges, then proceed in even smaller steps. Be guided by the child's actual performance, *not* by what you think or suspect he must be capable of doing.

Warnings. Some people are opposed to certain aspects of the systematic use of reinforcers with children, and this is especially so for the tangible reinforcers such as tokens, candy, or toys. In the course of your work with the child, his parents, and teachers, you may be called upon to justify your use of tokens or other reinforcers. It is best to anticipate their possible questions or objections so that you can make a good case for the treatment program you propose using. With this objective in view, let us now consider several of the most frequently voiced criticisms of the systematic use of reinforcement procedures. You might also wish to consult O'Leary, Poulos, and Devine (1972) for a more extended consideration of these issues.

1. *Criticism.* Reinforcement procedures are insensitive and mechanical, and will transform children into mindless automatons.

Reply. Competently conducted reinforcement programs are by their very nature extremely and continuously sensitive to the performance of the child. Their application is highly individualized and far from mechanical (see the description of shaping, Part 3 of this chapter). A therapist's insensitivity or rigidity will lead to failure of the program. Furthermore, contingency management is a tool, not an end in itself, and can be used in the service of a variety of values. Contingency management can be used to increase docile, passive behaviors in children displaying undesirably high rates of disruptive behavior, or it can be used to increase assertiveness and speech volume in quiet, withdrawn youngsters. Reinforcers can be administered for routine academic skills such as correct spelling or for independent and original efforts. For instance, teachers have employed reinforcement programs to increase the creativity of children's artwork (Goetz and Baer, 1973) and of their classroom performances (Reese and Parnes, 1970). Others have increased children's use of descriptive adjectives in conversational speech (Hart and Risley, 1968) and the quality of their creative writing (Maloney and Hopkins, 1973). As the Krasners (1973) and O'Leary (1972) have aptly pointed out, the behavioral approach describes certain laws governing human behavior and specific techniques for changing behavior, but does not dictate the goals for behavior change. Specification of desirable behaviors is a complex, social decision in which the behavior modifier is merely one participant.

Moreover, behavioral techniques can be employed flexibly in educational programs of great diversity including open as well as traditional classrooms (Krasner and Krasner, 1973) and individualized as well as group instruction (Keller, 1968). Rather than being impersonal and mechanical, successful reinforcement procedures are highly personalized, and can be used in the service of a multitude of goals.

2. *Criticism.* Reinforcement teaches children to work for extrinsic rewards, not for the sake of the activity itself.

Reply. In part, this is simply a pragmatic question. Take the case of the child who derives no intrinsic satisfaction from schoolwork or household chores. No amount of moralizing about the intrinsic satisfaction to be obtained from engaging in these apparently distasteful tasks is likely to persuade the child. The caretaker has his choice between standing on principle while the child fails to do the work or using reinforcement and shaping procedures to induce the child to engage in the desired activity. All too frequently, however, the adult issues moral injunctions as he punishes the child for failure to comply. The unfortunate result is that the schoolwork becomes even more aversive to the child as a result of its association with punishment.

A slightly different version of this objection raises a potentially serious issue, however. Some recent research indicates that one must be cautious about administering tangible reinforcers, such as prizes, for activities children have previously actively pursued without receiving special, extrinsic rewards. Lepper, Greene, and Nisbett (1973) have found that young children who were initially observed to display high rates of play with particular drawing materials (felt-tipped "magic markers") greatly reduced their subsequent use of these materials after they had been offered and had received a "Good Player Award" for using the pens in a brief training session. In contrast, children who neither were offered nor received an award did not reduce their later classroom use of the pens, nor did children who learned that they would receive the award only after they had finished the training activity. Because this is only an initial study, we do not yet know the conditions under which this effect will or will not occur. Under most circumstances, a therapist would not initiate a program to reinforce a child for a preexisting high-rate performance. Nevertheless, we must be alert to the possibility of undermining prior, naturally occurring maintenance conditions by imposing artificial reinforcement contingencies for previously well-established performances. The dangers posed may be most severe in situations in which the therapist has insufficient time available at the end of his intervention to wean the child from frequent, tangible reinforcers to very intermittent social ones. The gradual phasing out of the special reinforcers would probably permit the desired performance to continue under normal home or classroom conditions.

3. *Criticism.* But won't the performance simply collapse when the therapist leaves and the program is discontinued?

Reply. This can be a problem with any type of treatment intervention. The sudden, unplanned cessation of a therapy effort can indeed result in a return of problem behavior. This is why the best programs include a gradual transition from frequent, artificially imposed reinforcement to intermittent, naturally occurring reinforcement. At the same time, the administration of the training effort is transferred from the therapist to the child's family and to the child himself. In Chapter 9, we describe some of the methods for accomplishing such transitions.

4. *Criticism.* The child's classmates and siblings will see that he is receiving special treats and privileges while they are not. Won't the other children act up or complain about this unfair treatment?

Reply. Of course you must make sure that the disparity in treatment is not too great and that the children understand that the target child is receiving rewards for acting desirably, not badly. Various methods have been used to prevent deleterious effects on peer observers. Some therapists have administered the token reinforcers to the child at school and have arranged for the parents to provide the back-up reinforcers privately at home. This procedure prevents classmates from observing the target child receive his special reinforcers. The drawback to such an approach is that the parents may fail to follow through, and so the system may collapse.

Another procedure arranges for the target child to earn reinforcers for his entire class or for his siblings as well (see Walker and Buckley, 1972). O'Leary et al. (1972) caution that should the child fail to earn the reinforcer for the other children, they might harshly criticize or badger him. While this negative effect has not been reported to occur, it might well take place in situations the therapist cannot observe such as those on the playground or after school. This approach, therefore is also not foolproof.

Perhaps the most straightforward solution, and one also recommended by O'Leary et al. (1972), is to explain frankly to the children that the treatment is intended to help the target child with a particular problem he is having, and that his improvement will make life more pleasant for all of them.

Recent research (Christy, 1973) has indicated that imposing a reinforcement contingency providing edible reinforcers for individual children will have, if anything, a positive impact on the behavior of classmates. In a small special education class for preschool youngsters with behavior problems, Christy reinforced individual children for remaining in their assigned seats during a clay modeling activity. She found that while some of the other children initially commented or complained mildly about the target child's receiving the treats, they did not begin to misbehave or to act aggressively. In fact, some of the children began to remain in their own chairs more, at least initially. The teacher responded in a matter-of-fact manner to the children's complaints or comments about the target child's receiving the attractive rewards. She simply remarked, "I've got a deal with (child's name) now." Under these circumstances, at least, administering even highly prized edible treats such as marshmallows and nuts to a particular child failed to have harmful effects on observing children. Whether this result will also be obtained with other target behaviors, with older children, and with larger classes remains to be investigated. But these initial results are quite encouraging.

5. *Criticism.* This reinforcement system will turn children into conniving bargainers unwilling to do the slightest thing unless they are paid for it.

Reply. This sounds like the employers' familiar complaint against organized labor, doesn't it? But one could undoubtedly produce such an undesirable state of affairs with children by ill handling. Here again a forthright statement to the child should prove helpful. You explain to him that he earns rewards by doing things that are difficult for him, not for the easy things that he's been doing for a long time. Joke with him, and let him see how silly it is for him to ask for treats in exchange for simple jobs, and the incident will pass quickly. Be pleasant but firm. Remember that the overly manipulative child has been trained to act that way by adults who have acceded to his unreasonable demands.

These, then, are some commonly posed questions and criticisms concerning the use of tangible reinforcers with children. As we have seen, some of these objections are based on ignorance and are easily dispelled by a presentation of behavior principles or research results. Other objections contain at least a kernel of truth, and these require consideration in our treatment plans. The imposition of a treatment program is a matter of judgment. Do the anticipated benefits clearly outweigh the possible risks? Only good sense and careful deliberations can answer this key question.

Probe Questions for Part 2, Chapter 5

1. State Premack's Differential Probability Principle, and describe how one might use it in the interest of a child who refuses to go to bed at his bedtime.

2. Define each of these terms: reinforcing event, conditioned reinforcer, generalized conditioned reinforcer.

3. How would you establish a poker chip as a conditioned reinforcer for a four-year-old girl who likes to watch television?

4. Describe three methods for reducing the possibility of the child's becoming satiated with a reinforcer.

5. Why should a reinforcer be administered immediately after a desired behavior occurs? Give examples of reinforcers that can and those that cannot be administered immediately.

6. Suppose you had your choice between using a primary reinforcer (such as food), a simple conditioned reinforcer exchangeable for food, or a generalized reinforcer exchangeable for many different back-up reinforcers. Which of the three would you use in a treatment program and why?

7. State and reply to the most common objections to the use of tangible reinforcers with children.

Behavioral Objectives for Part 3, Chapter 5

When you have studied Part 3 of this chapter, you should be able to:

1. Devise a program to shape some new performance in a child.

2. Cope with extraneous behavior and performance cessation.

3. Detect the probable causes for a low rate of desired performance and institute a program to remedy the situation.

Part 3. Shaping and Strengthening Low-Rate Performances

Suppose now that a clinician is faced with the task of increasing the rate of some deficit behavior that the child has never before exhibited. What training methods are available? The therapist might choose to employ a shaping technique consisting of reinforcing successively closer approximations to a desired final performance. Alternatively, he could demonstrate the particular behavior himself and verbally instruct the child to imitate his example. Most often, however, the therapist will use a combination of demonstrations and verbal directions as prompts, and will reinforce the child for successive approximations. This and the following sections will discuss the amelioration of behavior deficits by means of shaping, and prompting by means of physical assistance, demonstrations, and verbal instructions. We will also consider the procedures used in remediating behavioral deficits in which the performance is infrequent but not unprecedented. In this latter circumstance, the deficit might be due to setting events or to inadequate cueing or reinforcement for the desired behavior. The type of intervention to be used depends upon the source of the child's behavior deficit.

SHAPING

Shaping is often used to teach new behaviors that the child has not previously performed. Shaping consists of the therapist's requesting and reinforcing successive approximations to the final behavior. Despite the popularity of the method and its simplicity in theory, the effective use of shaping techniques remains an art. One must select an appropriate initial performance requirement, must elicit and immediately reinforce correct behavior, must know when to proceed to a more stringent requirement, must choose an appropriately gradual succession of requirement levels, and must know how to deal with partial or total performance loss.

In order to shape a new performance through the method of successive approximations, it is necessary to have available a powerful, immediate reinforcer (Skinner, 1953). Timing is crucial in the shaping process. You must reinforce the desired approximation immediately, as any delay in reinforcer administration might cause some other intervening behavior to be strengthened. For example, you may wish to reinforce a child's sitting at his desk as an initial approximation to his studying his homework. If he approaches his desk and sits down, you must reinforce that act without delay. If you are not quick at it, he may begin to get up again. If you present him with praise or candy at this point, you will have inadvertently reinforced standing up rather than sitting down. Older children to whom you can explain the reinforcement contingency, or those who have experienced the contingency repeatedly, can often tolerate some delay between the performance and the reinforcer without the contingency's losing its effectiveness. But it is safest to assume that any delay will reduce the power of the manipulation.

As has been mentioned previously, conditioned reinforcers can usually be administered more quickly and flexibly than can such other reinforcing events as consuming food or candy, riding a bicycle, watching a television program, or staying overnight at a friend's house. Therefore, shaping procedures often involve the use of conditioned reinforcers. In the following example, the presumed conditioned reinforcers – praise and physical contact – are employed to teach a young child self-help skills. Note that these reinforcing consequences can be administered easily and immediately after the desired performance. Since dispensing them does not require much time, the reinforcement procedure does not interrupt or delay the course of the shaping process.

Example of Shaping

Let us consider the case in which the desired terminal performance for a young child is dressing himself in the morning. If might be necessary initially to place his legs in his underpants and only require him to draw the pants up to his waist, then give him praise and a hug. The second step in the shaping process might involve placing one of his legs in a pant leg and requiring him to insert the other leg before pulling up the pants and receiving reinforcement. When this performance has stabilized, the requirement might be for the child to complete the entire procedure by himself (see the sample program in Table 5-1).

Table 5-1 Sample Program Including a Shaping Procedure: Training a Child to Dress Himself

Step 1. Child's legs are inserted into his underpants. Underpants are drawn up to his knees. Contingency: Child must draw underpants up into wearing position in order to receive hug and praise (probably conditioned reinforcers). He is verbally requested to do so (prompt).

Step 2. Child performs Step 1 consistently (near 100%) upon request. Now only one of child's legs is inserted into underpants. Contingency: Child must insert other leg, then draw pants up to receive a hug and praise.

Step 3. Child performs Step 2 consistently upon request. Now he is required to pick up underpants, insert both legs, and draw pants up to receive positive consequation (hug and praise).

Step 4. Child consistently puts on underpants upon request. Now he is required also to put on slacks. [Note: In this and in each succeeding step, positive consequation follows successful performance.]

Step 5. Putting on a pullover shirt. The shirt is put over child's head; he must locate the sleeves, insert his arms, and pull down the shirt.

Step 6. Child picks up pullover shirt, pulls it over his head, locates sleeves, inserts his arms, and pulls shirt into place.

Step 7. Putting on socks. Socks are placed over child's toes. He must pull them up over his ankles. Shoes are put on him.

Step 8. Child must pick up socks, gather each one together, put it over his toes, and pull it up over his ankle. Shoes are put on him.

Step 9. Putting on shoes. Child puts on socks, shoes are placed before him in correct arrangement, right shoe in front of right foot. He must slip his foot into the shoe. Shoes are buckled or tied for him.

Step 10. Shoes are not placed before child. He finds shoes and puts them on the correct foot.*

***Note:** If this sounds like a difficult and tedious process, the description is correct. Winter weather in a cold climate further complicates matters by requiring boots, hats, mittens, and snowsuits. Even adults may have difficulty in outfitting themselves for excursions in subfreezing weather.

Guidelines for Shaping

The motto to adopt in shaping is to think small. Set your requirements at each stage at just what the child can master without too much strain. It is best to keep reinforcement density high; our experience is that the child should be earning reinforcement on 80 percent or more of his attempts to perform the desired behavior. Avoid long intervals during which the child receives no reinforcement because this will place many of his behaviors on an extinction schedule and he may cease trying. One way to avoid this possibility is to give the child some unearned reinforcers to help keep him working during the early phases of the program. An unearned reinforcer is one for which the performance requirements are either very minimal or absent. Its function is to maintain an activity level sufficient for shaping at a time when, for some reason, the child continues to emit incorrect, unreinforceable performances. Because they are not made contingent upon an acceptable approximation, unearned reinforcers must be used sparingly, but they occasionally prove very helpful.

The timing of closer approximations to the final performance is also critical to the success of a shaping program. Do not progress to a more stringent performance requirement until the child can consistently perform the behavior required at the preceding step. It is pointless to attempt to require the child to pick up his underpants and insert both legs if, having accomplished this, he only pulls the pants up to his waist successfully 50 percent of the time.

It is necessary to consider all possible reasons for a child's failure to meet a performance requirement. Perhaps he did not initially learn the easiest way to insert his leg into the underclothing. It may be that he was trying to do this while standing unsteadily on one leg. If so, you might suggest that he sit down to get his leg into his underpants, then have him stand up in order to pull them on. You might also have to demonstrate this operation for him yourself and give him considerable verbal instruction when he attempts it. Or you might offer him some physical assistance, help him keep his balance, and guide his hand or leg (physical prompts). Finally, you can ask him to put his foot into the leg hole and pull up the garment in order to earn his reinforcer.

Set specific criteria for reinforcement. Develop specific criteria for reinforcement for each step in the shaping program (see example in Table 5-1). Detailed criteria enable you to remember the precise nature of the reinforceable response at each stage in the program so that the child does not get reinforced for more distant approximations. If you reinforce indiscriminately, he will respond indiscriminately. Unless the performance is deteriorating and you need to drop back and restabilize an earlier performance, do not reinforce a poorer performance than that called for at the step at which the child is working.

How to deal with backsliding. Now suppose, in the example just mentioned, the child is consistently pulling up his underclothes. You then increase the requirement to Step 2: only one of the child's legs is inserted into the pant leg. He is required to insert the other leg, then draw the pants up. But, upon contacting this new contingency, his behavior breaks down, and you find that he neither puts his leg in nor pulls the pants on. What should you do? Return to the earlier requirement of his only pulling the pants on;

stabilize this performance once again, then reintroduce the leg insertion requirement.

In general, if a performance breaks down upon introduction of a particular contingency (e.g., Step 3), return to the preceding step (Step 2), and restabilize that performance. Then (a) introduce special cueing or prompting if that seems necessary, or (b) reduce the requirements at the next step (Step 3) so that the child can meet them more easily. Demanding too great an increment in performance can result in extinction not only of the required performance but also of preceding performances. Just remain flexible and let the child's behavior dictate the contingencies you set for him.

Performance cessation. If the child suddenly stops emitting correct responses, even though no new requirement has been introduced:

a. Go back to an approximation the child can emit without error, stabilize his performance, then increase your criteria more gradually and in smaller steps.

b. If this does not work, the child may have become fatigued or satiated on the reinforcer. Go back to a response the child can make successfully, reinforce him, and conclude that training session. Do not conclude a session with the child's repeated failure to perform correctly. End with a reinforced response so that the sessions themselves do not become aversive.

Extraneous behavior. In order to begin quickly shaping the desired behavior, it may be necessary incidentally to reinforce another, perhaps somewhat undesirable response if it occurs at a high rate and concurrently with the desired response. Perhaps a child is kicking the table strenuously and repeatedly while he is saying the required "puh." At the inception of training, it may be preferable to ignore the kicking, since it does not actively interfere with the desired vocalization. By not dealing specifically with the kicking, you will actually be reinforcing it because it occurs at the same time as the reinforceable verbal response. The kicking can be overlooked initially and dealt with if necessary at some later time when the child's verbal behavior has improved. Note that you would not want to reinforce highly undesirable acts that actually compete or interfere with the desired response. (In the example just cited, it might be best simply to move the table out of kicking range if that is possible.) The following chapter on excess behaviors will describe several procedures for reducing persistent disruptive behavior that interferes with the shaping process.

Application of shaping. Shaping procedures are frequently used to teach children complex skills not previously in their behavioral repertoires. Wolf, Risley, and Mees (1964) employed a shaping technique to teach a three-and-one-half-year old, highly oppositional boy to put on and wear the eyeglasses that were necessary for the preservation of his vision. Dickie, who has become a famous if not notorious child because of this widely read paper, not only refused to wear his glasses but would not permit anyone else to touch his head or put the glasses on him. Once the glasses were in place, he would tear them off and hurl them to the floor, frequently shattering them. This seemed to be an insuperable problem.

The experimenters originally planned to have the shaping procédure carried out by a ward attendant, to use candy as a reinforcer, and to begin with empty eyeglass frames in order to minimize breakage. None of these plans worked, probably because the attendant was not sufficiently skilled in shaping and the candy was not a sufficiently potent reinforcer for a non-food-deprived child. Modification of the eyeglass frames so that they fit like a cap made the task much easier for the child, so the treatment could proceed at once with his putting on and wearing prescription lenses.

A skilled therapist, rather than a ward attendant, conducted the training. Clicks from a toy noisemaker were established as conditioned reinforcers followed by Dickie's receiving bites of food. To enhance the potency of the food reinforcer, his regular meals were withheld, and food was made contingent upon his correct performance. First, he was reinforced for picking up and holding any of several pairs of empty eyeglass frames, which were placed around the room. After he reliably approached and held the glasses, he was required to bring the frames closer and closer to his eyes in order to earn reinforcers.

Dickie was successively reinforced first for placing the earpieces straight over his ears, and then for also looking through the lenses. His looking through the lenses was also prompted by the experimenters' displaying interesting objects for him to view, such as a ring or the clicker.

In the last phases of training, Dickie was required to wear his glasses in order to participate in appealing activities such as taking accompanied walks, going to the playground, taking automobile rides, eating snacks, etc. Whenever he took off his glasses, the activity was terminated. At the completion of the program, Dickie was wearing his glasses for about 12 hours each day.

This case study not only informs us about a successful shaping endeavor, it also illustrates some of the difficulties therapists might encounter. Applying the shaping procedure through a second agent, the aide, proved time-consuming and ineffective, so the authors were forced to intercede and carry out the program themselves. Although they did establish a conditioned reinforcer (a click), the child's food-satiated state made the candy first offered him a weak and fragile reinforcer. The experience of Wolf, Risley, and Mees, then, underscores the importance of managing the shaping process yourself, except in unusual circumstances. It also points up the futility of attempting to use as reinforcers stimuli for which the child has not been deprived, a consideration we discussed in a preceding section on choice of reinforcers. Further, it should be noted that Dickie's highly oppositional behavior and his lack of an imitative repertoire necessitated the lengthy shaping procedure described here. With a child who behaved less deviantly, the therapist could have demonstrated the proper use of eyeglasses and verbally directed the child to wear them; thus, the difficult and time-consuming shaping process could have been considerably abbreviated.

STRENGTHENING LOW-RATE PERFORMANCES

Sometimes a behavioral deficit consists not of the total absence of a particular desired behavior but of its occurrence at an abnormally low rate. Suppose the child has at some time engaged in the desired behavior – for example, washing the dishes – but that he does so only very rarely. Probably no lengthy and complex shaping process is required in this instance, but the situation must be analyzed to determine the reasons for his low performance rate. Consider the components of a functional analysis of behavior – setting events, antecedent stimulus events, the target behavior itself, and consequent events. The reason for a low rate of performance may lie in any one or more of these factors. Since the child in our example actually does display the target behavior on occasion, a shaping process appears unnecessary. Perhaps setting events make the desired performance unlikely. It could be that the boy is tired at dishwashing time after a day of schoolwork, active play, and a large dinner. Perhaps the dishwashing chore deprives him of the opportunity to watch his favorite television program or to play with his friends who are having a noisy ballgame outside the window. If these are the reasons for his failure to help with the dishes, a possible solution might be to change his chore time. The dishes could just be stacked in the kitchen after dinner to be washed at some later, more convenient time. Or the family's dinnertime might be changed to an earlier hour to avoid scheduling conflicts with his favorite pastimes. Possibly his work assignment might be changed from dishwashing to setting the table and helping with food preparation so that he would be free after dinner. Good behavior therapists can typically generate a number of different possible solutions; if a particular intervention proves unprofitable or not feasible, another can be introduced.

Concerning antecedent events, perhaps no clear signal is given the child regarding the proper time to start washing the dishes. Sometimes he is expected to begin before laggards have finished their dinners, but on other occasions he must wait until all have finished. Sometimes the completion of the dessert course is the cue, but at other times he is allowed to leave the table and watch television for a while until his mother's insistent instructions signal him to begin cleaning up. Under such circumstances, no one event reliably sets the occasion for the child to begin his work, and his performance is understandably unreliable. His work routine might be more easily established if the last diner's putting his napkin on the table were the stimulus event that nearly always preceded dishwashing time.

The youngster's cleaning work also might be facilitated by the provision of models, such as another family member's beginning to clear the table or wipe down the kitchen work surfaces. His father might offer a prompt such as, "Let's get these things off the table and washed up so that we can all go out for an ice cream cone," and might begin handing the dirty dishes to his son to aid in the clean-up.

Let us suppose that the setting events and antecedent events all favor the successful completion of the desired act. The child is neither overly fatigued nor deprived of some attractive competing activity. The cues to engage in the target behavior are clear, reliable, and unequivocal. The physical circumstances may place limits on the child's performance. He might be too short to reach the sink easily, or the work space might be otherwise very inconvenient for him, requiring undue exertion on his part. A simple rearrangement of the work area or provision of a stepstool may solve a major portion of the problem. Another source of the deficit may be motivational. What reinforcers are available to strengthen and maintain the child's performance? Perhaps members of his family all go their separate ways, gratefully, while he is left alone with a pile of dirty dishes – not too attractive a prospect. The reason for a low performance rate, then, may lie in inadequate reinforcement. The reinforcers offered may be too small in magnitude (just an occasional smile from mother), too infrequent (once or twice a month), or both, so that naturally the child does not respond positively to his parents' requests. To remedy this situation, the parents might come into the kitchen with him to chat, play guessing games, read poems and stories, or otherwise entertain and reinforce him while he does his work. If this is not feasible, the child might be paid for finishing the dishwashing, or he might receive both money and parental attention for his efforts.

As we have seen, a child's behavioral deficits can spring from a variety of possible sources. Modification programs that employ several types of interventions are more likely to be successful than are attempts that focus only upon any one set of possible determinants such as reinforcing events. It is, of course, much more difficult to identify the effective components of such complex interventions (see Part 4 of Chapter 4), but they do have the advantage of being more likely to produce dramatic improvement than programs that manipulate only the reinforcement schedule.

Since your primary goal is to produce positive change, you will probably choose effectiveness over elegance of analysis. So long as there remains some way of assessing the effectiveness of the particular treatment program employed, however complex that program is, one can satisfy both the evaluational and the therapeutic requirements of applied child behavior analysis.

Probe Questions for Part 3, Chapter 5

1. What should you do if a child's previously stable and predictable responding breaks down upon introduction of a more stringent performance requirement?

2. In which of the following situations should the child be given an unearned reinforcer and why? (a) Daisy is being taught to imitate some simple movements, such as clapping, but she stops watching the therapist and looks out the window. (b) Robert is attempting to zip his parka (the required performance), but repeatedly gets the cloth caught in the zipper teeth.

3. What are the advantages of generous reinforcement of children's performance attempts during shaping?

4. Describe how Dickie was taught to wear glasses. What difficulties arose and how were they overcome?

5. Suppose that a child only rarely obeys his teacher's instructions. What potential determinants of this behavioral deficit should be considered in designing a treatment program.

Behavioral Objectives for Part 4, Chapter 5

When you have studied Part 4 of this chapter, you should be able to:

1. Plan and carry out a shaping program involving the use of conditioned reinforcers, prompts, and the fading of prompts.

2. Incorporate therapist demonstrations of desired behaviors into training programs, when applicable.

3. Decide when instructions should be used in therapeutic programs.

4. Devise instructions appropriate for use with children.

5. Fade instructional prompts so that naturally occurring stimuli gain control over the target behavior.

Part 4. Prompting Deficit Performances: The Use of Physical Guidance, Modeling, and Instructions

PROMPTING

If the child never or only very rarely emits the desired behavior, and if you attribute this low rate to a deficit repertoire rather than to inadequate incentives, use instructions, modeling of desired responses, cueing, prompting, or putting through (sometimes called passive shaping) so that the behavior will occur and can be reinforced. If you are attempting to teach the child to say a "puh" sound, for example, you would model the initial approximation by saying "puh" to him several times, then you might prompt him on the sound by holding his lips together while he attempts to spit, and reinforcing him after each appropriate attempt. When he says "puh" reliably with the aid of the prompt, start fading the prompt. Instead of holding his lips in place, you now just touch his lips. When he has mastered this stage, then just hold your fingers to his chin. At last you can take your hand away and he is still successfully saying "puh."

Other prompts you might use include explaining how to position the lips or tongue to produce the sound, or you could exaggerate the necessary motions or sounds as you demonstrate them for the child. Table 5-2, a portion of a language development program developed by Jane Y. Murdock and Barbara Hartmann (in press), lists prompts frequently used in speech training.

As another example of a prompt, therapists who wish to teach a child to maintain eye contact with them and who are using food as a reinforcer frequently employ the following procedure. The therapist holds a spoonful of food up to his face near his eyes and instructs the child, "Look at me." Since the food is attractive to the child, he looks at it and, in the process, looks the therapist in the eye. As soon as the child responds correctly to the command, "Look at me," the prompt of holding the spoon up is faded, and the performance is under appropriate stimulus control.

The prompts you use should not be negative or coercive in tone. For example, a good way to prompt the sound "Mm" is to dip a popsicle stick or tongue depressor in some good-tasting liquid like honey and pop it into the child's mouth while asking him to say "Mmmm." Remember to keep your prompts as pleasant as possible.

Other prompts that have been successfully used include the teacher's placing a preschool youngster in a chair to prompt appropriate sitting (Twardosz and Sajwaj, 1972), giving a simple verbal direction such as "Stand up" and a sufficient gesture or actual tug to insure the child's correct response

Table 5-2 Illustrative Procedures for Training Expressive Language Skills (from Murdock and Hartmann, in press)

Category II: Phonological (Sounds) Skills

Discriminative Stimuli (Instructor)			Response (Child)	(2) Consequent Stimuli (Instructor)
(3) Verbal	Visual	(1) Prompts to be used if needed		
1. "Say (sound)" 2. "Say (sound), (name of child)" 3. (sound) 4. (sound), (name)	Instructor's face	1. Physically place child's mouth in initial position for sound. 2. Physically touch part of mouth important to production of the sound. 3. Tell child how to form sound with tongue, lips, etc. 4. Say the sound with the child. 5. Visually and auditorily exaggerate sound. 6. Visually exaggerate your facial movements unique to sound.	Correct imitation of sound or gradual approximations to correct sound.	Reinforce 1. CRF Social CRF Tangible 2. CRF Social FR2 Tangible 3. CRF Social VR5 Tangible
			Incorrect response	No reinforcer

Note: For each task as the child reaches one of the defined criteria, (1) fade prompts, then (2) thin reinforcement schedule, and (3) change verbal discriminative stimuli appropriate for the next task in this category. Move to next number in *each column* after child gives ten consecutive correct responses or responds correctly 80 percent or better for two consecutive sessions.

in teaching self-help skills to retarded girls (Minge and Ball, 1967), and taking the child's hand and putting it through an action requested such as pointing to his nose, picking up the cup, or clapping his hands (Whitman et al., 1971). These types of prompts are quite commonly used in childrearing, and can be useful in initiating correct behavior. Unfortunately, many caretakers and children become reliant on these types of physical guidance, and continue to use them long after the child could have been performing the act unassisted. The prompt must be removed gradually, as is described in the next section.

Fading prompts. Fade prompts in small steps and as quickly as possible while still maintaining correct performance. If you fade too slowly, the child may perseverate at some step and you might have to turn to some quite different performance in order to get him learning again. For example, perhaps you have been trying to teach the child to say "Mama," and despite your best efforts to shape him to say the whole word, he continues to say "Maaa." The best course of action might be to drop the training of "Mama" temporarily and begin to work on another word ("Hi"), then return to the word "Mama" at some later time. This may prevent an impasse from developing.

If you fade prompts too quickly, the performance might break down. In this latter case you must return quickly to an approximation the child can perform and start building again from there. An example of the systematic fading of prompts is offered in O'Brien, Bugle, and Azrin's (1972) account of training a profoundly retarded child to eat with a spoon. The child was provided with a bowl of food, which was in the form of a lumpy paste. Initially, the teacher provided manual guidance as follows:

> (1) The handle of the spoon was placed in the child's right hand. (2) Guiding the hand, the spoon was dipped into the food, and with food on the spoon, it was lifted to about 1 inch above the bowl. (3) The spoon was lifted to within 2 inches of the child's mouth. (4) The teacher placed her left hand on the child's chin and gently opened the child's mouth. (5) The spoon was gently guided into the child's mouth. (6) The child's hand was guided upward and outward resulting in the food being removed from the spoon by the child's upper teeth or lip. (O'Brien et al., 1972, p. 69)

At first the teacher guided the child through all six of the steps. Evidence of stability of performance was followed by the elimination of a prompt. Thus, whenever the child completed the sequence correctly on three successive assisted trials, the teacher guided her through one less step on the next assisted trial. In each instance, the prompt omitted is the terminal one in the behavior chain, the one temporally closest to reinforcement. Note that rather than eliminating a number of prompts abruptly, just one is dropped at a time. The performance is again stabilized through three successive correct trials, then one more prompt is dropped, and so on until no prompts are used.

On the other hand, whenever an assisted trial was not completed correctly, the trial was interrupted and another guided trial was begun, which included one additional step. In this manner, the amount of prompting or guiding done by the teacher was continually adjusted in accordance with the child's performance at any given time (see O'Brien et al. [1972] for additional details). There is no formula for devising and programming prompts, so you must monitor the child's performance very closely and add or delete prompts accordingly.

Modeling

In many instances, both modeling and demonstrating and physical guidance prompts are used (Bandura, 1969). For example, in teaching fearful children to approach nonpoisonous snakes, Ritter (1968) successfully used exposure to fearless peer models who handled snakes and gentle physical guidance to lead the child to touch and handle a snake. This training method proved to be highly effective.

Speech training programs frequently employ both the therapist's modeling of the desired sounds and physical prompting to help the child produce the sound (Sloane and MacAulay, 1968). In teaching the sound "f" to a child, the therapist may say, "Johnny, say 'f.'" If the child does not respond correctly to this instruction and modeling procedure, the therapist may then light a candle and have the child blow the flame in order to prompt the "f" sound. In speech training it is often possible to proceed efficiently without such nonverbal prompts, but as Bandura (1969, Chapter 3) has pointed out, it is virtually impossible to teach language without recourse to modeling. In normal speech development, children are exposed to millions of examples of appropriate speech usage, and their own attempts at imitative speech quickly become functional in the acquisition of reinforcers. Similarly, in more formalized speech training, the therapist must demonstrate the target vocalization if the training program is to progress efficiently.

In some instances, such as in the training of aggressive behavior, provision of relevant behavioral models may suffice to increase an observer's rate of aggressive responding. Shaping or reinforcing the observer's behavior may not be necessary as long as his aggressive acts are not punished (Bandura, Ross, and Ross, 1963; Christy, Gelfand, and Hartmann, 1971; Hicks, 1965; Nelson, Gelfand, and Hartmann, 1969).

Modeling alone has also been found effective in increasing the frequency of the use of descriptive adjectives by young children enrolled in a Head Start program (Lahey, 1971). When an adult model used descriptive adjectives (e.g., of color or number) in talking about a set of toys, the children subsequently employed adjectives in their own comments about other toys, although they had not previously used adjectives nor were they explicitly reinforced for doing so.

Modeling procedures have also been found to enhance social interactions in socially withdrawn nursery school children (O'Connor, 1969). The children were shown a 23-minute film depicting youngsters engaging in a graduated sequence of interactions ranging from very calm to vigorous interactive play. A narrative soundtrack described and praised the filmed models' behavior. Although no response consequences were provided the subjects, those who observed the modeling film subsequently engaged in more social interactions than did those who viewed a control film depicting dolphins performing tricks.

These two studies demonstrate that children who display minor behavior deficits can significantly benefit from exposure to exemplary models even though the children are not differentially reinforced for imitation. Of course, in the long run, reinforcing outcomes are necessary at least intermittently in order to maintain the behavior. In therapeutic programs that aim at producing the greatest behavioral change in the shortest amount of time, generous reinforcement of desired responses is usually provided.

When to use modeling. When should you incorporate modeling procedures in treatment programs? Obviously, modeling as well as physical prompting techniques are helpful whenever the rate of the desired behavior is near zero. A rare behavior affords few reinforcement opportunities, and therefore shaping may proceed very slowly or not at all (Bandura, 1969). If a child never says any sounds resembling those in the word "baby," a shaping process alone would prove tedious and unreliable. Modeling and prompting are virtually required.

When a child emits a high rate of undesirable behavior, provision of models performing a competing, appropriate behavior can also be an effective modification technique. For example, if a child almost invariably responds to interpersonal conflicts with aggressive and domineering behavior, provision of successful, cooperative models may encourage attempts at cooperative acts (Chittenden, 1942), which can then be increased and maintained through reinforcing consequences.

Similarly, provision of successful models is important whenever the results of erroneous performance are highly unpleasant or dangerous. Thus, you would not rely solely on a shaping procedure to teach a child how to light a gasoline camp stove. You would first demonstrate how to operate the stove, then monitor the child's attempts in order to forestall a potential disaster. And, as Bandura (1969) has also pointed out, very intricate but not dangerous performances such as learning the sequence of movements in a dance, necessitate the provision of appropriate models. Consequently, most treatment programs aimed at increasing deficit behavior (and many of those designed to decrease behavioral excesses) will employ modeling procedures.

Instructions

Unlike his colleague who works with animal subjects, the modifier of human behavior has at hand rapid methods for prompting desired behaviors. Pity the animal trainer. Anyone who has witnessed experimental psychology students fruitlessly shouting advice to a recalcitrant rat learner in an experimental chamber is easily convinced of the utility of verbal instructions in prompting performances of appropriate (human) subjects. The more fortunate clinician can demonstrate a particular behavior pattern to his client and can verbally instruct the client to emulate his example. If he has previously learned to imitate appropriate models and to follow instructions, the learner need not be subjected to a lengthy shaping process. The therapist might merely state, "Watch me build a block tower [and demonstrate the process]; now you build a tower just like mine." Under favorable circumstances, the child quickly complies, even though he may never before have worked with these particular play materials. This child has probably previously been reinforced for obeying adults' requests, so that instructions have acquired discriminative properties and set the occasion for his compliance (Skinner, 1957). If the child is verbally skilled and has also had the relevant construction experiences, the therapist's symbolic verbal model, "Can you build me a tower using these five blocks?" should suffice to elicit the requested performance.

Although one could use an unprompted shaping procedure to train the child to construct the tower, this alternative would probably prove more stressful and time consuming. First the child would be reinforced for approaching the blocks, next for picking one up, and then (perhaps after some length of time and repeated trials and errors) for piling one on top of another. Considerable further time might pass before the child would pile another block on top of the first two. In the meantime, both trainer and child might suffer from inadequate reinforcement for their efforts.

Since the combination of example and instructions provides the most information most quickly, such teaching procedures are frequently used. You should take advantage of whatever imitative and verbal skills your child-client demonstrates. If he can follow instructions, use them. If he frequently imitates adults, demonstrate what you wish him to do. And, of course, you will want to reinforce his correct attempts.

Limitations. The situation is not always that straightforward. Occasionally one runs across a child who simply does not obey most instructions. He may not have been reinforced for obedience or he may have been accidentally reinforced for disobeying adults' instructions. Perhaps whenever he complied with a request from his parents, they ignored him, but his disobedience resulted in some type of reinforcing interaction with them. Naturally, instructions do acquire discriminative properties for this child – but for his noncompliance rather than his obedience.

Such a process has been documented in research studies. Both Bucher (1973) and Hopkins (1968) have found rapid decreases in instruction-following in the absence of explicit response consequences for compliance. In other words, a good way to train a child to disobey is to issue numerous commands but not reinforce him for obeying them. In fact, Madsen, Becker, Thomas, Koser, and Plager (1968) have found that a teacher's repeated instruction "Sit down!" resulted in an increase in children's *standing up* when compliance was not differentially reinforced. In contrast, children's conformance with instructions has been reliably increased by the provision of positive consequences such as social attention (Schutte and Hopkins, 1970; Zeilberger, Sampen, and Sloane, 1968), tokens exchangeable for back-up reinforcers (Baer, Rowbury, and Baer, 1973; Zimmerman, Zimmerman, and Russell, 1969), or a combination of approval and tokens (Bucher, 1973). Baer et al. (1973) also found that a combination of token reinforcers for compliance and a one-minute timeout (during which the child was seated on a chair away from play materials) effectively increased negativistic preschool children's responsivity to teacher instructions. It would appear advisable in working with an oppositional child first to increase his rate of instruction-following, and subsequently to teach him other social skills. Compliance with instructions seems to constitute a generalized response class similar to generalized imitation (Bucher, 1973; Whitman et al., 1971). Therefore, it is usually not necessary to train the young child to comply with a particular request if he has previously learned to follow adults' instructions and can perform the requested behavior.

Instructions can also facilitate responsiveness to reinforcement contingencies. In an experiment conducted with adults, Ayllon and Azrin (1964) found that verbally instructing adult psychotic inpatients to pick up eating utensils and reinforcing them for doing so resulted in greater appropriate cutlery usage than did either instructions or reinforcement contingencies alone. Under some circumstances, then, verbal instructions can significantly improve therapeutic effectiveness. For this reason, we advocate their use, but with the precautions described next.

Guidelines. Instructions are likely to prove most effective if they are carefully phrased. One should remember in working with young children that their vocabularies are limited as contrasted with the verbal facility of adults. Suggestions made to young children should be unambiguous, consistent, and intelligible to the child. It is inadvisable to say to a six-year-old, "Just perform a modicum of academic work, and your parents will accompany you to the cinema." These instructions are imprecise (what is a modicum, what kind of academic work is required, and what movie will they see?). And the vocabulary required to understand this statement is probably far beyond that possessed by a young child. The child's response to such an instruction is likely to be either, "What did you say?" or an uncomprehending smile and nod. In either case, the therapist will have a lot of explaining to do.

A second guideline is that the instruction be phrased positively as a suggestion or invitation rather than as a peremptory command. The direction, "Clean up your desk" sounds both harsh and uninviting as opposed to, "As soon as everyone has cleaned up his desk, we can leave for our trip to the zoo." Not only does the latter statement seem less like an order, but it also presents a pleasant inducement for compliance. And then there is the incidental modeling effect to be considered. Children may attend to and exhibit not only the behavior symbolically modeled in the directive (e.g., to clean the desk) but also the manner in which the instruction is presented. Adults who have fallen into the habit of barking orders to children are not infrequently dismayed to overhear the youngsters in turn shouting rude commands to others. So it is to the child's advantage to witness adults making reasonable and pleasant suggestions, but not continuously.

Fading Instructional Prompts

Since it is advisable to set up a variety of nonverbal stimuli as discriminative for desirable behavior, instructions are ordinarily discontinued after their initial application. For example, it is more appropriate and far safer to have the sight and sound of the roadway and of passing vehicles become discriminative for a child's looking in both directions before proceeding across a street than for his mother's instructions to be the only signal that he should behave cautiously. So, while instructions can be helpful aids early in the training process, overreliance on instruction can impede performance. You should tell the child about the contingencies you have set up, but don't nag him into compliance or he will come to respond to nagging rather than to more appropriate cues for action.

The same procedures used to fade reliance on physical prompts for the required performance can also be used to fade the issuing of instructions. As the child practices the correct action, the verbal instructions issued by the caretaker become increasingly telegraphic and infrequent as other cues – such as the time of day – acquire discriminative stimulus properties. For example, a mother might initially make considerable use of instructions in training her child in a bedtime routine. The instructional interchange might occur as follows:

SITUATION. A mother is using instructions to help teach her five-year-old son to brush his teeth and put on his pajamas in preparation for bedtime. He performs both tasks upon request, and his mother wishes him to do so without her having to remind him.

TIME. First evening through fourth evening of training.

Mother: "Roger, it's bedtime. Now brush your teeth and change into your pajamas, then we can read your story book." (She reinforces Roger for obeying by praising him and reading to him.)

TIME. Fifth evening.

Mother: "Roger, bedtime. Remember what to do?"

Roger: "Oh yeah, tooth brush time."

Mother: "Right; then into your jammies and hop into bed." (She then reinforces Roger for complying.)

TIME. Sixth evening.

Mother: "Remember what to do at bedtime, sweetie?"

Roger: "OK, brush those teeth, get into jammies, and nighty-night."

Mother: "That's my big boy! Then I'll read to you before lights out."

TIME. Tenth evening.

Mother: "Roger, time to get ready for bed." (Roger goes into bathroom, brushes his teeth, walks to his bedroom, changes his clothes, and climbs into bed. Mother then enters bedroom.)

Mother: "Good boy. What shall we read tonight?"

Note that in the preceding sequence the mother has progressively decreased the complexity and length of her instructions until at last no mention of tooth-brushing or clothes-changing is necessary. Those behaviors have come under the control of one simple instructional statement that bedtime has arrived.

To summarize, verbal instructions can be helpful ingredients of therapeutic training programs if they are used to provide information on behavior consequences or to inform the child of desirable response alternatives. Instructions should not become the sole cue for many desired performances lest the child become overreliant on them. To prevent inappropriate dependence on instructional cues, one can limit the use of verbal instructions to the initial portion of a program, or can greatly abbreviate them over the course of training.

Gradually omit instructions as the child's performance comes increasingly under the control of other, more convenient and appropriate situational cues.

Probe Questions for Part 4, Chapter 5

1. Give examples of physical prompts that might be useful in teaching a child to ride a tricycle.

2. How can a therapist prevent a child from becoming overreliant on physical assistance prompts?

3. Under what circumstances can modeling be used without explicit reinforcement procedures but still effectively to remove a behavioral deficit? Give examples.

4. What purposes do instructions serve in child behavior modification programs? When might instructions prove counterproductive?

5. Why is it desirable to fade or decrease the issuing of instructions as a child becomes more practiced at a desired target behavior?

Behavioral Objectives for Part 5, Chapter 5

Study of Part 5 of this chapter should enable you to:

1. Write and implement a performance contract with a child and his caretakers.

2. Prepare a written script describing all aspects of the treatment program.

Part 5. Contingency Contracting and Preparing a Treatment Program Script

CONTINGENCY CONTRACTING

One of the best ways to engage the child in the behavior modification project and to assure his cooperation is to set up a contingency contract with him. This contract spells out clearly and concisely the amount and type of work on his part, and the amount and type of reinforcer he will receive. A written contract is sometimes drawn up and signed by both the child and the therapist so that the reinforcement contingencies to be employed are clearly understood and agreed to by both parties. A sample contract appears in Table 5-3. As compared with merely spoken contingency agreements, the written contract provides greater clarity and specificity. It may also produce a greater commitment to behavior change on the part of the child. Moreover, the contract discourages capriciousness in the contract manager's work demands and in his reinforcer distribution.

The written contract additionally provides a convenient vehicle for a transition from behavior management by other persons (therapist, teachers, parents) to self-contingency management or self-regulation by the child client. For example, Homme, Csanyi, Gonzales, and Rechs (1970) suggest a succession of steps leading from complete manager control of work requirements and reinforcement contingencies to complete client self-control of contingencies. When the child's behavior comes predictably under the control of the manager-determined contract, the transfer to self-control can begin. In the first phase, the child is given some voice in determining the type and amount of required performance and reinforcement. The child and manager either jointly determine the amount of task performance required and the child alone determines the reinforcer, or the child alone decides the work requirement and they jointly determine the amount of reinforcement. The child is systematically given practice in specifying work requirements and reinforcer allocation, and he is additionally reinforced for doing so. As the child becomes more accomplished in setting up his own reinforcement contingencies, the manager's role fades until at last the child has assumed sole control. We will reserve our consideration of other self-control training procedures for a later section of this manual (see Part 2 of Chapter 9).

Table 5-3 A Sample Contingency Contract to Increase Studying

I, (child's name) , agree that I will do the following work, for which I will get the rewards specified:

1. Study the subject (s) (math and spelling) in (my bedroom) and no other place.*
2. Begin studying at (7:00 p.m.) and stop studying at (7:30 p.m.) and (do at least 2 pages of math problems and study my spelling list once.)
3. Report accurately the amount of schoolwork I do at home each day.
4. Study these subjects each day assigned: (Mon., Tues., Wed., Thurs., Sun.)
5. For my work, I will get the following rewards:
   a. (A dessert of my choice at 8:00 p.m.)
   b. (To select the television program the family watches at 8:00-9:00 p.m.)
   c. (To attend a Saturday afternoon movie of my choice.)
   d. ______
   e. ______
6. I will also receive (5 ¢) for (each problem sheet returned by the teacher with 80% correct) and (50 ¢) for each (spelling test on which I get at least 90% correct).
7. For each week I do all the work described, I will also (be allowed to invite a friend to Saturday lunch and movie).
8. But if I claim one of my rewards without having earned it, I will be fined (75 ¢).

______________________________(Child's Signature)

______________________________(Manager's Signature)

**Note:* Fox (1962) advocates establishing effective stimulus control over studying by setting up one particular time and place uniquely related to study, and where incentives for engaging in competing behaviors are minimized.

Lloyd Homme and his associates (Homme et al., 1970) have devised a set of rules to guide the novice in contingency contracting. They are as follows:

"Rule 1. The contract payoff (reward) should be immediate.

"Rule 2. Initial contracts should call for and reward small approximations.

"Rule 3. Reward frequently with small amounts.

"Rule 4. The contract should call for and reward accomplishment rather than obedience." (*Note*: This rule represents a value judgment on Homme's part, but one with which we agree. It is, however, not based upon empirical evidence. The principle is that the child should not become overly dependent upon the contingency manager.)

"Rule 5. Reward the performance after it occurs." (In other words, do not give the reinforcer to the child *prior to* his performing the specified responses.)

"Rule 6. The contract must be fair." (This is a stickler. It implies that you must be careful to see that you have the child's genuine agreement to the contract, and that you have not intimidated him into agreeing to terms that he cannot really accept.)

"Rule 7. The terms of the contract must be clear." (Each party should know explicitly what is expected of him and what he can expect in return.)

"Rule 8. The contract must be honest." (No welching allowed on either side.)

"Rule 9. The contract must be positive." (There is some difference of opinion on this point. Homme prefers that the contract offer something positive to the child, over and above that which he can expect in his everyday experience, and that the contract include no threat of punishment or deprivation. In practice, many contingency managers write in response-cost clauses for the child's falsifying records or otherwise cheating on the contract. Stuart [1971] maintains that a good behavioral contract should include a system of sanctions for failure to meet responsibilities outlined in the contract. Stuart, in work with adolescent delinquents, finds that on occasions in which the teenager might find it more reinforcing to violate the contract than to give up the promised reinforcers, the sanctions may tip the balance in favor of compliance with the terms of the contract. But, in general, contracts do accentuate the positive.)

"Rule 10. Contracting as a method must be used systematically." (Homme, et al., 1970, pp. 18-21). (Do not reinforce undesirable behavior; be consistent. Perhaps when you are rushed or are feeling tired, you might neglect to reinforce a desired response as called for in the contract or might allow an undesired response to go unconsequated. Or you might just forget to pay the child at the conclusion of an agreed-upon work interval. If his contracted performance breaks down, it will very likely be due to the unsystematic use of contracting.)

As an additional consideration, Stuart (1971) suggests the incorporation in the contract of a bonus clause that offers additional amounts of positive reinforcement for some extended period of near-perfect compliance with the terms of the contract. Here, again, the availability of the extra incentive may help outweigh the reinforcers to be gained by violating the agreement. So you might want to offer the child extra points or money, or entertainment privileges for one or two weeks' compliance with his contractual responsibilities.

A written contingency contract can play a useful role in child behavior modification in that it increases the commitment of the participants, it clearly specifies the obligations and the advantages to all, and it does not lend itself to misunderstanding, capriciousness, or distortion due to faulty memory so much as does a conversational agreement. Whether or not you elect to use a written contract, you will want to prepare a script describing your treatment program, a topic we consider next.

THE WRITTEN PROGRAM

Because precision and consistency are essential to the success of a behavior modification program, it is advisable to prepare a written script describing each detail of the setting, the equipment, and the procedures used. The written script helps insure that all therapists are following the same procedures in their work with the child, and that each therapist does not change his practices midway through the program because of errors of memory. The script also helps remind the therapist of the materials he must have on hand for each treatment session. Another advantage is that the written program can be incorporated into a final project report as the description of the modification procedures employed.

Table 5-4 presents a format you might use for writing up your treatment program. In addition to the categories presented in Table 5-4, you might wish to include procedures designed to promote generalization of prosocial target behaviors (see Chapter 9). It would also be helpful to include your plans for phasing out and concluding your work with the child. Many treatment agencies appreciate receiving a copy of your treatment program so that they can continue the training effort after you have left the agency. Your making the program available is a distinct benefit to the agency and to the child-client, especially if the program was effective.

Table 5-4 Treatment Script Format

I. *Objectives.* This portion of the written program describes the anticipated terminal behavior produced by the treatment intervention. Example: At the completion of this program, Alice will engage in a normal amount of interactive play with other children. Specifically, at least 60 percent of her play time will be spent in interaction with children. (The required percentage would be based upon observations of the percentage of interactive play engaged in by peers.)

II. *Acquaintance Procedures.* Describe how you will become acquainted with the child prior to initiation of the treatment program. Example: The therapist will have lunch with the child two times and will take the child for a walk through the park.

III. *Setting.* Describe the location and times at which the modification program will be carried out. Example: The training sessions will occur in an individual tutoring booth at 10:00 a.m. each weekday morning.

IV. *Materials.* Provide a list of materials that the therapist should have on hand for each session. Example: picture stimuli, paper tissues, cereal and soft drink reinforcers, data recording materials including clipboard, data sheets, pencil, stopwatch.

V. *Data Collection.* Describe how the behavior will be scored and recorded. Example: On the prepared data sheet, the observer will enter a check mark in the proper box for each 10 sec. interval Johnny spent in studying. For each training session, the observer will calculate the percentage of intervals during which Johnny studied. This figure will be entered on Johnny's graph.

The baseline data collection procedures should also be described here. Example: Johnny and his teacher were instructed to follow their usual procedures for his schoolwork. An observer recorded his study behavior in the classroom during the reading period at 10:00 to 10:45 a.m. each morning.

Moreover, a schedule for the collection of reliability data throughout the program should be included in the script. Example: Interobserver reliability checks will take place on the third session during each phase of the program.

VI. *Modification Program.* This is the script the therapist will follow in conducting training sessions with the child; it should be complete enough to allow some other person to carry out the same program independently.

a. *Session Length.* State how long each session will last and how often sessions will occur. State criteria for concluding a session (e.g., if the child begins making errors on material previously mastered, if he appears very bored or restless after having been eager and attentive). Include instructions on how to conclude the session (e.g., return to a performance the child emits successfully, reinforce that performance, and conclude on this positive note).

b. *Reinforcers.* Identify and gain control over reinforcers. If necessary, establish conditioned reinforcers (describe how this will be accomplished). For token reinforcers, specify where and when they will be exchanged for back-up reinforcers and describe the back-up reinforcers.

c. *Reinforcer Delivery.* Specify when the reinforcers are to be delivered to the child, and by whom. Example: After each vocalization that follows the therapist's vocalization within 5 sec., the therapist will praise the child and give him one poker chip token. Also state the reinforcement schedule to be employed and the criteria to be used in thinning the reinforcement schedule. Example: Reinforce every correct response until the child reaches a criterion of 90 percent correct response (or some other near-perfect level) for at least two consecutive training sessions.

d. *Modeling and Prompting.* Specify the modeling and physical prompting methods to be used, if any. Example: The therapist instructs the child, "Do what I do. Now clap you hands." The therapist demonstrates, then takes the child's hands and claps them together. You must also describe when and how the prompts will be faded.

e. *Shaping.* If you are using a shaping procedure, describe the steps to be used in performance requirements and the criteria for proceeding to each closer approximation. Example: When Billy pulls on his shoes successfully 90 percent of the time when requested to do so, require him to pull the straps through the buckles.

f. *Reviews.* Describe the schedule to be followed in reviewing previously mastered performances. Example: Review all previously mastered performances at least once during each session. Intersperse review trials with new tasks so that the child has just successfully completed a review item prior to the introduction of a new requirement.

g. *Competing or Disruptive Behaviors.* State the procedures to be used in dealing with the child's disruptive behaviors. Example: Whenever the child begins to get up from his chair or look around the room or squeal, the therapist will sit quietly looking away from the child until the child sits down and attends to the therapist. Then the therapist begins the next training trial.

Probe Questions for Part 5, Chapter 5

1. Describe the advantages of formalized, written performance contracts as compared with informal conversational agreements.

2. What types of information are typically included in contingency contracts?

3. How might one use a contingency contract to train a child in self-regulation?

4. Discuss the probable consequences of violation of each of Homme's rules for contingency contracting.

5. How will the preparation of a treatment program script benefit the therapists, the child, the child's caretakers?

6. What types of information should be included in the treatment program script?

Behavioral Objectives for Part 1, Chapter 6

After you have finished reading this section, you should:

1. Be aware of the professional ethical principles governing the use of aversive behavior control techniques.

2. Know the considerations governing the choice of a response reduction technique.

3. Be able to state the conditions under which an extinction procedure will be maximally effective.

4. Be able to describe the possible side effects of extinction procedures.

5. Be able to describe a DRO procedure and its merits relative to simple extinction.

6. Know when and how to use discrimination training.

CHAPTER 6

Reducing Excess Behaviors

Part 1. Ethical Considerations, Extinction, DRO, and Discrimination Training

Deceleration interventions present a number of problems over and above those encountered in acceleration programs. For instance, it is important to realize that there are very few occasions on which it is desirable only to decelerate a given behavior without at the same time training the child in some alternative prosocial act. In other words, it is rarely desirable to employ a deceleration program alone. This is so because you ordinarily do not want to reduce the net total of reinforcement the child is receiving. A behavior that is eliminated is not generally replaced by *no* behavior. It may be replaced by some other performance that might be equally undesirable if you do not take pains to see that the child learns a socially appropriate alternative behavior. Laboratory findings also indicate that there will be a greater suppression of a punished response when the child is provided with an alternative response that will earn him reinforcement than if no such alternative is offered (Azrin and Holz, 1966; Herman and Azrin, 1964; Holz, Azrin, and Ayllon, 1963). This effect may also hold for deceleration techniques other than punishment. For example, a DRO (differential reinforcement of other behavior) procedure may eliminate an undesired performance faster than would an extinction procedure alone.

ETHICAL CONSIDERATIONS

The use of aversive control techniques requires responsible, professional judgment. The therapist must be quite certain that the target behavior actually requires modification and that aversive control techniques are the method of choice. Sometimes it is the caretaker's rather than the child's behavior that merits alteration, but the actual situation is not obvious at first glance since the caretaker is the complainant. For example, a parent may report that her child is disobedient and hyperactive, while on closer examination it turns out that it is the mother rather than the child who is behaving deviantly. In one such instance, Bernal, Williams, Miller, and Reagor (1972) found the child to be acting quite normally, but his mother was imposing undue restrictions on him and was issuing commands to him at the rate of up to nearly 300 per hour. Presumably, this atypical maternal behavior would have been discovered by a behavior therapist during the initial assessment and baseline observation phases of a treatment project. Instances such as this one do point up the need for very careful assessment of the situation, especially where unwarranted punishment might be meted out to a child. If the parent's expectations and behavior are deviant (rather than the child's), it is the responsibility of the therapist to acquaint the parent with normative data on child behavior, and perhaps for him to arrange to have the parent observe other children and parents in an effort to alter the unrealistic parental perception of the child.

Of course this must be accomplished as tactfully as possible if it is to prove successful. In such circumstances, you should consult with your instructor before approaching the child's parents. Your instructor may help you to formulate a plan for overcoming the child care agent's defensiveness and for aiding the child. Or, if your instructor concurs, it might be advisable to refer the family to an experienced professional practitioner for longer term guidance.

Before you embark upon an aversive control program, it is also helpful to hold a group discussion with your instructor and classmates to consider a number of alternative treatment strategies. When you are faced with the problem of controlling a high-rate, annoying target behavior, it is frequently easier to devise some punishment procedure than to generate a pleasanter and perhaps even more effective positive control method such as reinforcing a competing behavior. Since punishment also sometimes produces undesirable behavioral side effects, which we will discuss later at some length, a positive behavior manipulation tactic is often to be preferred. As compared with solitary decision making, the group discussion promotes a more complete consideration of the advantages and disadvantages of a contemplated deceleration intervention.

Before proceeding to a description of the various deceleration techniques, we will take a moment to review some professional ethical principles that relate to treatment procedure choice. We urge you to employ these principles in your work. The guidelines offered here are based upon the American Psychological Association's *Ethical Principles in the Conduct of Research with Human Participants* (1973), which contains the following statement regarding the use of physically or psychologically stressful procedures:

> The ethical investigator protects participants from physical and mental discomfort, harm, and danger. If the risk of such consequences exists, the investigator is required to inform the participant of that fact, secure consent before proceeding, and take all possible measures to minimize distress. A research procedure may not be used if it is likely to cause serious and lasting harm to participants. (p.2)

The Ethical Principles also contain warnings against exposure of "susceptible participants," especially children, to research involving physical discomfort or danger. It is argued that children may be more frightened and upset by painful experiences in part because they may be less familiar with them. Further, since children are less physically and socially powerful than adults, they are relatively defenseless participants whose "fundamental trust might be violated" by undue exposure to stress (American Psychological Association, 1973, p. 65).

It is recognized, however, that the use of procedures involving physical discomfort may be more warranted when the participant could derive some direct benefit, as in a therapeutic situation. Concerning therapy, the Principles state:

> Although the diagnostician or therapist should be cautious in the use of dangerous procedures, even for the patient's benefit, it may be reasonable to tolerate a higher likelihood of adverse effects when the treatment is being employed for the possible benefit of the participant than when it is being employed strictly for research purposes. (p.66)

Nevertheless, the clinician must use great caution, particularly when working with children.

In general, it is good ethical practice to restrict the infliction of pain to circumstances in which no effective alternative treatment methods are available, and the child's guardians have given their fully informed consent. You must have considered any negative side effects in advance and must be prepared to deal with them should they arise. You should not engage in any procedure that will leave the child worse off than before treatment.

We urge you not to employ any potentially harmful stimulus (such as electric shock, which could prove lethal in the hands of amateur electronic technicians) or other corporal punishment. You are responsible for having thorough knowledge of the procedures and any equipment you use and of any potential hazards associated with its use. It is good practice to expose yourself to any noxious stimulation you intend to employ so that you become quite aware of the unpleasant aspects of experiences to which you subject others. In all treatment questions, your primary duty is to insure the welfare of your clients.

CONSIDERATIONS IN SELECTING DECELERATION TECHNIQUES

Several different deceleration methods can be used; the choice among them depends, in part, on whether the reinforcer maintaining the objectionable behavior can be identified. If you know or have a very strong suspicion of the identity of the maintaining reinforcer, you can use an extinction technique or can systematically reinforce alternative behaviors and put the deviant behavior on an extinction schedule (DRO). If you have little idea of what factors control the target behavior, it may be necessary to use a punishment procedure. If the reinforcer itself is undesirable or inappropriate for the child, a satiation procedure may be in order. Each technique has advantages and disadvantages, which we will discuss in some detail. The considerations governing the choice of a deceleration technique are summarized in Table 6-1.

Extinction

The term extinction is applied to a procedure in which reinforcement that has previously followed an operant behavior is discontinued. No restraint is used to prevent the child from performing the behavior, but, when he does so, he no longer receives the reinforcer. Under extinction procedures, the previously reinforced behavior generally decreases in rate, perhaps following a temporary rate increase (extinction burst). If the maintaining reinforcer has been identified, extinction procedures can be used. You must gain control over the dispensing of the reinforcer and consistently withhold it following the undesired behavior. This is easy in principle but difficult in practice. It implies that not only you but all of the people with whom the child comes into contact must withhold reinforcement for that particular behavior. Unless the child is institutionalized or is an infant, it is difficult to achieve the necessary control over his social environment.

When to use extinction. The optimal situation in which to use an extinction procedure is when the target behavior has previously been consistently reinforced. When the response has been maintained on a near continu-

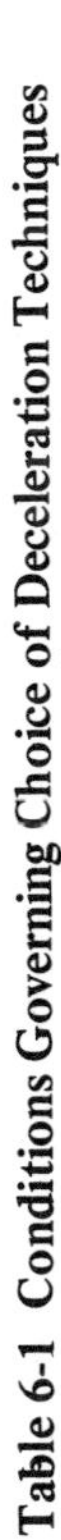

Table 6-1 Conditions Governing Choice of Deceleration Techniques

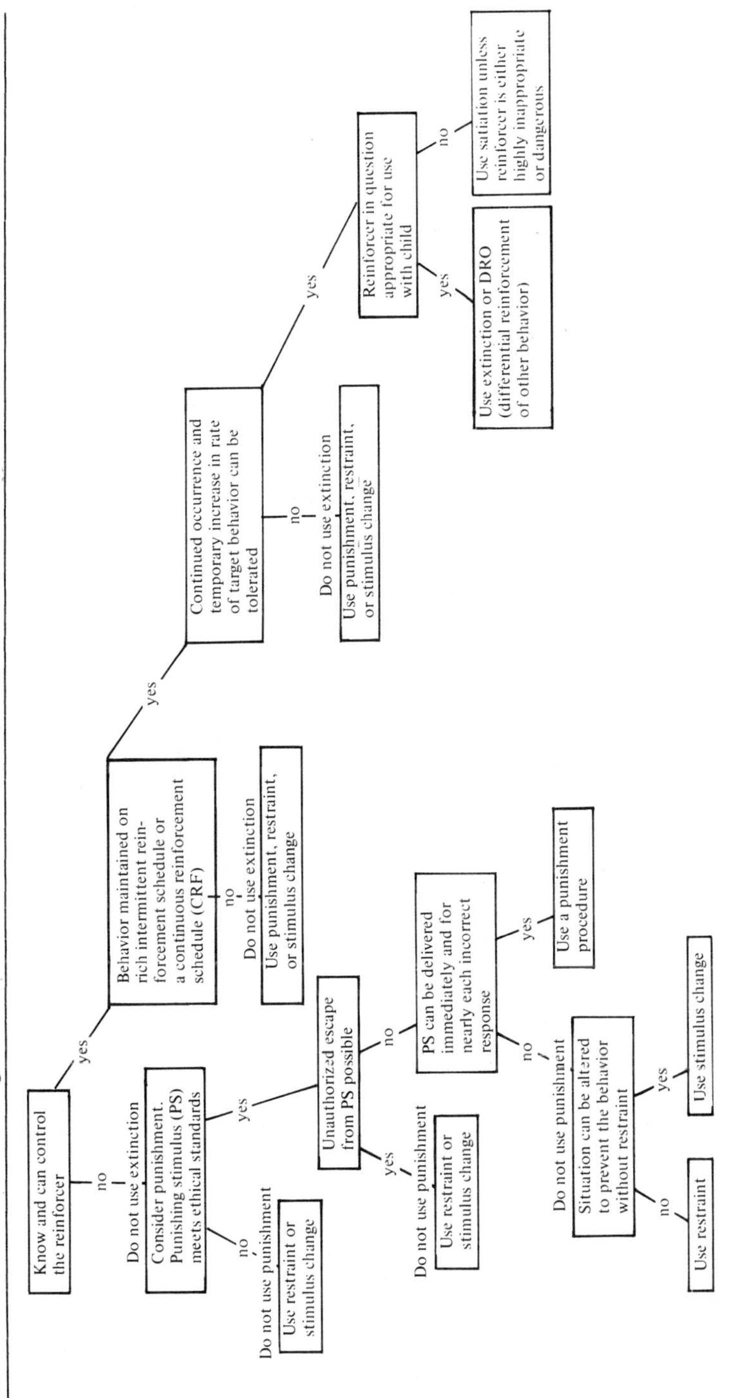

ous reinforcement schedule, the extinction procedure is easily discriminated by the child and takes effect most rapidly. The process can be very slow if the target behavior was maintained on a lean intermittent schedule. It might be some time before the child discovers that no more reinforcement is forthcoming for the target behavior, and the resistance to extinction of behaviors maintained on intermittent schedules is a well-documented phenomenon (Ferster and Skinner, 1957).

Also, as mentioned previously, if extinction is to be used, it must be used consistently. The reinforcement must be withheld completely and over a long period of time in order to eliminate a particular response. Half measures are doomed to fail. Indeed, parents frequently report that they have tried an extinction procedure on their child's misbehavior, but that it did not succeed. In fact, the misbehavior got worse. What has often happened in such cases is that the parents had encountered a transitory increase in the rate of the behavior just put on extinction. Since they were unprepared for the temporary increase in rate of the target behavior, they mistakenly concluded that their modification procedure was not working and abandoned it prematurely. Suppression of behavior does not occur immediately with extinction, so that this technique is not desirable for use with dangerous responses (e.g., firesetting, extreme aggression, self-mutilation) that cannot safely be ignored by caretakers (Risley, 1968; Tate and Baroff, 1966).

Side effects of extinction. If you are using an extinction technique, be prepared for a temporary increase in the rate of the target behavior at the inception of extinction. It is well to prepare the child's caretakers to expect behavioral fluctuation. Assure them that this will be temporary if everyone persists in keeping the misbehavior on an extinction schedule. You might also observe emotional behavior in the child and some increased variability in his rate and type of behavior. The emotional behavior can be reduced somewhat if you have arranged for the reinforcement of an alternate, competing response and have informed the child of the new conditions under which reinforcement is available. There are conditions under which the attempted, systematic use of extinction procedures by parents and teachers has proven ineffective (O'Leary et al., 1969; Wahler, 1969; Wahler, Winkel, Peterson, and Morrison, 1965). Alarmingly, in other instances, carefully controlled experimental studies have found differential caretaker attention for prosocial behavior and ignoring of deviant behavior (attempted extinction) to result in dramatic increases in the rate and severity of some types of misbehavior (Herbert, Pinkston, Hayden, Sajwaj, Pinkston, Cordua, and Jackson, 1973; Sajwaj, Twardosz, and Burke, 1972). In none of these instances, however, was caretaker attention established to act as a reinforcing event for the highly oppositional, disruptive children observed. Consequently, it was possible that removal of the parent's or teacher's attention following the deviant behavior did not actually constitute extinction because adult attention was not the reinforcing event maintaining the misbehavior.

In several of the instances reported, the children's undesirable behaviors were subsequently successfully controlled through the imposition of a classroom token reinforcement program (O'Leary et al., 1969), a timeout procedure (Wahler, 1969; Wahler et al., 1965), or a combination of teacher attention for appropriate behavior and timeout for disruptive behavior (Sajwaj et al., 1972). These results indicate that unless adult attention has been definitely identified as a reinforcer for the child, and attention can be reliably withheld following deviant activities, some other response elimination technique may be preferable to extinction.

In summary, an extinction procedure is effective in reducing the rate of undesirable behavior, but it is difficult to apply. You must be able to eliminate all sources of reinforcement for the target behavior and you must persist in your procedure until you have achieved success. It is best if the target behavior was previously maintained on a CRF schedule. If you can meet these requirements, extinction may be your deceleration technique of choice.

Applications. Harris et al. (1964) and their colleagues have used extinction techniques most successfully in controlling various misbehaviors on the part of nursery school children. These investigators not only extinguished a particular undesirable behavior (such as whining and crying) through withdrawal of teacher attention, but they simultaneously administered approving attention for the child's prosocial behavior incompatible with the misbehavior (Hart, Allen, Buell, Harris, and Wolf, 1964).

The general method employed consisted of identifying the reinforcer probably maintaining the undesired performance and then removing that reinforcer following the performance. Teacher attention was found to be the maintaining reinforcer for the children's inappropriate behavior, and removing contingent teacher attention controlled such various misbehaviors as regressed crawling (Harris, Johnston, Kelley, and Wolf, 1964), isolate play (Allen, Hart, Buell, Harris, and Wolf, 1964; Johnston, Kelley, Harris, Wolf, and Baer, 1964), and aggressive attacks (Brown and Elliott, 1965). In addition, infants' inappropriate, high-rate operant crying has been eliminated through extinction by the removal of caretaker attention (Etzel and Gerwirtz, 1967; Williams, 1959). In their study, Etzel and Gewirtz (1967) also reinforced the infants' smiling and eye contact with adults–actions incompatible with crying. It is notable that extinction procedures involving withholding of adult attention have usually proved successful with infants and nursery school-aged children and that the reported treatment failures have been with older children. It may be the case that adult attention is more likely to act as a potent reinforcer for very young children while older children respond to a wider variety of other reinforcing events.

DRO

In circumstances in which it is desirable to discontinue reinforcement for some excess behavior but is unwise to decrease the quantity of reinforcement the child receives, the therapist might choose to employ a DRO (differential reinforcement of other behavior) procedure. The DRO technique consists of differentially reinforcing any behavior *except* one specific target behavior. The target behavior is thus placed on an extinction schedule while behavioral alternatives are reinforced. For example, in attempting to reduce the frequency of temper tantrums in a two-year-old child, the child's play is observed and he is reinforced for any play behavior except tantrums. If he throws a temper tantrum, the normally forthcoming reinforcement is withheld. Presumably, his rate of verbal and physical outbursts will decrease, and his rate of alternative behaviors will increase.

A variation of the DRO procedure involves reinforcing just one class of actions that are themselves desirable and are incompatible with the targeted misbehavior. If the misbehavior consists of shouting rude commands to other children and adults, this misbehavior might be placed on extinction. At the same time, the child could be reinforced for speaking quietly and politely – an activity incompatible with screaming imprecations.

The DRO procedure is frequently applied in demonstrations of behavioral control resulting from differential reinforcement procedures. When the DRO contingency is put into effect, the target behavior's rate decreases if the reinforcement contingency used by the therapist was, in fact, responsible for the previous rate increase.

Advantages of DRO. The DRO procedure is relatively simple to use. All you need to do is specify a misbehavior, identify and gain control over its reinforcing consequences, and systematically withhold reinforcement for the misbehavior while consistently reinforcing either (a) any other action the child engages in, or (b) a specific, competing behavior. The latter alternative has the advantage of strengthening some particular class of prosocial activities while reducing the rate of the unwanted behavior. Both procedures are often more advantageous than either extinction alone or punishment in that the child's net rate of reinforcement received does not decrease. In fact, he may even get more reinforcers than he did before the DRO contingency was employed. Since he is not being deprived of his accustomed reinforcers, the youngster is less likely to protest the treatment program than if he experienced either simple extinction or punishment manipulations.

Discrimination Training

Sometimes a child may perform a response that is undesirable only because of the time and place of its occurrence. In itself, the performance may be essentially desirable. Only the circumstances are wrong. Example: the child talks and laughs with his friend, an appropriate behavior, but taboo while the teacher is addressing the class. In such an instance, you would want to train the child to discriminate between the appropriate and the inappropriate situations and to behave accordingly.

Implementation. Use every means at your command to make the appropriate (S+) and inappropriate (S-) situations as different from each other as possible (Terrace, 1963, 1966). The easier the discrimination task is made, the faster the child will learn the correct performance. Then the discrimination can gradually be made more subtle and difficult as the child continues his correct performing, until at last he is successfully using the cues normally present in his natural social environment. Returning to the case of the child who talks and jokes, but under inappropriate circumstances, you might have him wear some distinctive and attractive article of apparel (perhaps a special badge) during the time when he is supposed to be quiet and attentive, and then remove the article when he is free to talk with his friends. Any sort of noticeable but not disruptive cue can be used – an electric lightbulb, a sign, a flag, a hat, a necklace, or some other type of clothing. Then reinforce the child for responding appropriately, in this case for working quietly in class (and perhaps for joking with friends between classes). Remember to keep the discrimination task as easy as possible at first and to administer many learning trials.

You must be able to control all sources of reinforcement so that neither you nor anyone else reinforces the child for the target misbehavior in the (S-) situation. If necessary, arrange the environment so that it is very convenient for the child to emit the response under the appropriate situations and very difficult to emit it under the undesirable circumstances. Teachers frequently attempt to do just this by seating close friends some distance apart when classroom silence is necessary. The environmental barrier makes the incorrect response much more difficult to perform. Do not be punitive about it, but do make whatever rearrangements are desirable to facilitate correct performing. In addition, describe the reinforcement contingencies to the child to make sure that he understands that he will gain reinforcement only for correct discrimination performances.

Probe Questions for Part 1, Chapter 6

1. Why is it usually unwise to reduce the rate of an unwanted behavior without also teaching the child a socially desirable alternative behavior?

2. Under what circumstances would you *not* want to reduce the rate of a child's behavior that a teacher finds offensive?

3. Why should even more caution be used in applying a behavior reduction program than in a shaping procedure?

4. Describe the conditions under which it is ethically acceptable to expose a child to physically or psychologically stressful procedures.

5. What behavior deceleration techniques can be employed when the reinforcer maintaining the undesirable behavior can be identified? What techniques are appropriate when the maintaining reinforcer is unknown?

6. Under what circumstances would the use of an extinction procedure be counterproductive?

7. DRO and extinction: how are they similar, how do they differ, and what are the advantages and disadvantages of each?

8. Describe a procedure to teach a child to speak quietly while indoors and to shout and squeal only when outside.

Behavioral Objectives for Part 2, Chapter 6

After studying this section, you should be able to:

1. Define punishment and describe instances of the use of punishment procedures.

2. State the possible negative effects associated with the use of punishment.

3. Discuss the safeguards that should accompany the use of punishment.

4. Describe the conditions that will maximize the effectiveness of punishment.

5. Devise a response reduction program based upon a timeout procedure.

6. State why it is desirable to use brief timeout periods.

Part 2. Guidelines for the Use of Punishment and Timeout Procedures

A punishment procedure can be used even if you have not been able to identify the reinforcers maintaining the child's misbehavior. Punishment can be defined as the presentation of an aversive stimulus contingent upon the emission of a given response. Under optimal conditions, the punishment suppresses the target response either temporarily or permanently.* Parents frequently use punishment to discipline their children, but with varying degrees of success and sometimes complete failure (Sears, Maccoby, and Levin, 1957). In this section of the manual, we will describe the various punishment procedures and present guidelines for their use.

Following the practice of Azrin and Holz (1966), we will include timeout and response-cost consequences under the general heading of punishment procedures. Thus, in our usage, punishment could consist of making critical comments (e.g., "That was a naughty thing to do," or "You are acting like a monster."), presenting physically noxious stimuli (e.g., shaking, spanking, or clapping your hands loudly), programming timeout from the availability of reinforcement (e.g., isolating the child briefly), or assessing response cost contingent upon misbehavior (e.g., fining the child).

Some people so strongly oppose the use of aversive control procedures that they prefer not to explore the topic at all. Our position is the more moderate one of describing procedures in current use, but providing considerable cautionary information. We certainly do not recommend employing any such technique except with the greatest sensitivity to the rights and the welfare of the child involved. Moreover, any type of punishment procedure lends itself too readily to overuse and abuse, so it might be best employed as a last, rather than a first attempt to remedy either treatment or childrearing problems. One should recognize, however, that aversive control techniques differ greatly in intensity and acceptability. Some harsh techniques should perhaps never be used, while others are very mild, yet effective, and are frequently employed in naturalistic teaching and childrearing situations. For example, simple verbal prohibitions may suffice to lead children to desist from some inappropriate activities. Many people who oppose the use of corporal punishment with children do not find verbal prohibitions or other punishment

*There are a number of different definitions of punishment currently in use. Azrin and Holz (1966, p. 381), for example, prefer to define punishment in terms of its impact on behavior: "Punishment is a reduction of the future probability of a specific response as a result of the immediate delivery of a stimulus for that response." Other investigators (Church, 1963, p. 369) prefer to use the term to refer to a procedure rather than a behavioral effect: "the punishment procedure is one in which an aversive stimulus is contingent upon the occurrence of a response." There is no generally agreed upon definition at present.

methods objectionable. The corrective procedures of placing the child in isolation briefly or fining him for misconduct are generally considered acceptable if administered fairly and not over-used. Many parents and teachers do use these latter measures routinely and successfully with children in their care.

Sometimes a child engages in disruptive behaviors at a rate sufficient to interfere seriously with a shaping program designed to teach him imitation, object identification, speech, or some other necessary skill. In this frequently encountered circumstance, the therapist must somehow reduce the rate of disruptive behavior so that the child can learn new skills. The therapist's initial management procedures might consist of attempting to demonstrate, to physically prompt, and to reinforce appropriate sitting and attending behaviors incompatible with disruptive behaviors. Should these remedies fail, a second tactic is to attempt extinction of the unruly behavior by withdrawing therapist attention. If, despite this procedure, the child persists in his aggressive or inappropriate behavior or his escape attempts, a longer timeout period or a mild punishment procedure might be employed as described in the following portion of a language training procedure developed by Murdock and Hartmann (in press).

Procedures to Eliminate Inappropriate or Nonattending Behaviors

Attending is defined as sitting upright in the chair and looking at the instructor or other visual stimuli for 3 seconds or more.

A. If the child is not attending, verbalize instructions simply and clearly. Model the desired behavior. Physically place the child in the appropriate position and assist him in going through the desired behavior by guiding his arm toward his body or otherwise demonstrating precisely what it is that you want him to do. Caution should be used here to insure that you are not reinforcing non-attending behaviors by talking to or physically handling the child. Keep accurate data to determine whether correct responding is increasing with fewer prompts required. If not, the following procedures should be used.

B. Withdraw your attention from the child and do not attend to him until he has been attending appropriately for 3 seconds.

C. Take a reinforcer yourself, pairing it with the same social praise you would use with the child, e.g., "Very good sitting," etc.

D. If the child exhibits hand-in-mouth, hands-over-eyes, grabbing behaviors, etc., establish arm-folding or hands-in-lap behaviors before proceeding with the program. This may be done by modeling the behavior and reinforcing the child's correct imitation, or it may

> be necessary to physically move the child through the arm-folding or hands-in-lap behaviors, gradually fading out the physical prompting and reinforcing the child for each approximation to the desired behavior.
>
> E. If the child emits a high rate of a specific inappropriate behavior, present an aversive stimulus immediately following that inappropriate behavior, e.g., loudly verbalize, "No!" This may be paired with a sharp rap on the table, desk or chair or a loud hand-clap. (pp. 5-6)

Note that in the preceding program, the initial efforts are based on positive intervention techniques – only when these attempts fail are even mildly aversive consequences used. In addition, the most aversive procedure described involves only verbal reprimand and a loud noise. Such carefully graduated sequences insure that the therapist employs the least stressful procedures that prove effective in reducing the disruptive behavior to a level compatible with the child's participation in a shaping program.

Warnings. Punishment is a controversial behavior control technique and great care must be taken with its use (see the previous discussion of professional ethics). You must be sure to obtain the informed consent of the child's caretakers before embarking on a punishment program, and you must be sure that you have not overlooked the possibility of using alternative modification programs based on positive control principles. Some charges frequently leveled against punishment are that it can produce disruptive and undesirable emotional behavior, sometimes has an initial general suppressing effect on behavior other than the target behavior, produces avoidance of the punishing agent or aggression directed toward the punishing agent (Azrin and Holz, 1966), can produce elicited aggression against nearby and innocent bystanders (Ulrich and Azrin, 1962), and is sometimes effective only in the presence of the punitive agent (Risley, 1968) or only as long as the punishment procedure is in effect (Azrin, 1960). Additionally, it has been pointed out that punishing agents can serve as models for aggression, and that punishment can have the paradoxical effect of intensifying the very response it is designed to suppress, especially in the case of aggresive acts and of negative emotional expressions such as crying (Bandura, 1962). On the positive side, punishment has been used successfully to provide lasting suppression of undesired responses.

It is important to know and to guard against the negative side effects of punishment procedures. Good sources of information on punishment theory and research include Azrin and Holz (1966), Campbell and Church (1969), Church (1963), and Solomon (1964). Accounts of clinical use of punishment techniques are to be found in Bucher and Lovaas (1968) and Neuringer and

Michael (1970), and are reviewed in Bandura (1969), Bucher (1969), Gelfand and Hartmann (1968), and Kanfer and Phillips (1970).

Guidelines. Now let us suppose that the excess behavior poses a serious problem, that all positive control efforts have failed, and that caretakers and therapist are agreed that some aversive procedure is warranted. What conditions are necessary for the most effective use of punishment over the briefest period of time? Since stressful procedures should be used sparingly, if at all, it is highly desirable that the punishment procedure immediately suppress the problem behavior so that punishment can be discontinued as quickly as possible. Careful planning is necessary to achieve this goal. In their often cited review of punishment research, Azrin and Holz (1966) offer a number of suggestions for the maximally effective use of punishment. These authors suggest (Azrin and Holz, 1966, pp. 426-427) that if you attempt to eliminate a behavior by punishment, you should proceed as follows:

1. Arrange the punishing stimulus in such a manner that no unauthorized escape is possible. Your punishment procedure is not likely to meet with much success if the child can tune out your verbal reprimands, or if he can plug his ears to avoid hearing an aversive noise stimulus, or if he is contentedly watching TV while you think he is in timeout. He may go so far as to avoid you (the punishing agent) or the situation in which he is punished, so that he becomes a truant from school or home.

2. Make the punishing stimulus as intense as possible while still causing no physical damage. A large body of research indicates that more intense punishing stimuli are more effective than are weaker stimuli.

3. "The frequency of punishment should be high as possible; ideally the punishing stimulus should be given for every [incorrect] response." If you punish intermittently, the chances are that the misbehavior is being reinforced intermittently and will therefore become more resistant to control.

4. Deliver the punishing stimulus immediately after the response. Otherwise neither you nor the child can be quite sure what behavior is being punished.

5. Introduce the punishing stimulus at maximum intensity, do not increase it gradually. Gradual introduction can allow adaptation and significantly decrease the effectiveness of even a highly intense punishing stimulus.

6. Avoid extended periods of punishment, especially when you are using low intensities of punishment, since the procedure may cease to be effective. Azrin and Holz suggest confining the use of mild intensities of punishment to brief time intervals.

7. Take great care to see that the delivery of the punishing stimulus is not differentially associated with the delivery of reinforcement. This phenomenon is actually fairly common in everyday life. Suppose that a child mis-

behaves and causes his mother to lose her temper and spank him. The mother might be, and often is, overcome by guilt at her loss of control and tries to remedy the situation by showering the child with affection and reassurances that she really does love him. If this sequence recurs repeatedly, the mother's punishment can become discriminative for the ensuing reinforcement. One then finds the apparently paradoxical situation in which punishment results in an increase of misbehavior (Katz, 1971).

8. Reduce the degree of motivation to emit the punished response. The threat of capital punishment for stealing bread is not likely to deter a starving man. Feed him, and the threat of punishment becomes a more effective control technique.

9. Also reduce the frequency of positive reinforcement for the punished response. If the child's defiance of the teacher earns him the plaudits of his classmates, he will continue to defy the teacher despite relatively severe punitive consequences. If stealing yields highly valued items, the stealing may continue even though it is punished.

10. Make available to the child an alternative response that will not be punished but that will produce the same or greater reinforcement as the punished response. Thus, in reaction to the child's defiance of the teacher, a prosocial way of earning approval from the classmates (and the teacher) should be provided the child. Similarly, the thief might be given some job through which he can earn the money to buy the items he previously stole.

11. If no alternative response is available, give the child access to a different situation in which he obtains the same reinforcement without being punished. As an example, the overweight child who sneaks food from the refrigerator between meals and at night might be punished for doing that, but allowed free access to selected foods at mealtimes.

12. "If it is not possible to deliver the punishing stimulus itself after a response . . . [a] conditioned stimulus may be associated with the aversive stimulus, and this conditioned stimulus may be delivered following a response to achieve conditioned punishment" (Azrin and Holz, 1966, p. 427). The most common form of conditioned punishment is a verbal command such as "no" or "stop that," which accompanies a physical restraint or parental slap. After several such pairings, the verbal command acquires conditioned punishing properties and can effectively suppress misbehavior when presented alone.

Findings from laboratory research with children provide the basis for two more suggestions to guide contingency managers in the use of punishment:

13. Punish early in the child's transgression sequence rather than later or after the undesirable act has been completed (Aronfreed and Reber, 1965). It is particularly important to punish early if mild punishment is being applied

(Parke, 1969). Following this reasoning, one would punish a child when he is reaching for the crystal goblet, not after he has held it.

14. Inform the child of the reasons for his not engaging in the punished behavior. If the act is dangerous or harmful to his health, tell him so. If it is detrimental to others or is illegal, make sure that he understands that these facts provide the rationale for the punishment, not your personal whim or your desire to exert power over him.

Incorrect reason given for punishment:	"Because I say so, that's why."
Correct reason given for punishment:	"Because smoking can give you cancer or heart trouble and because it's illegal for a 12-year-old to buy cigarettes."

Considerable research evidence indicates that restrictions placed upon children's behavior (e.g., refraining from playing with prohibited toys) are more effective in the absence of the punitive agent when the child has been informed of the reasons behind the restrictions (Cheyne and Walters, 1969; Parke, 1969). See Parke (1970) and Walters and Parke (1967) for reviews of the effects of punishment on children's behavior.

Since timeout and response-cost procedures are generally less socially objectionable than physical punishment, they are the punishment techniques most frequently used in clinical work with children. Consequently, we shall describe these procedures in detail.

Timeout

In recent years timeout from positive reinforcement has come into increasing use as a response suppression procedure.* Nonavailability of positive reinforcement is equivalent to extinction; a timeout period is therefore a period associated with extinction, and it can serve as a punishing stimulus (Azrin and Holz, 1966). A timeout procedure differs from extinction as applied to a specific behavior in that no positive reinforcement is available for *any* behavior as long as the timeout is in effect. Descriptions of timeout techniques and the probable mechanisms by which they operate are available in Leitenberg (1965) and in Zimmerman and Ferster (1964). In clinical applications response-contingent timeout from the availability of positive reinforcement has been used to eliminate children's tantrums and aggressive behavior (Tyler and

*We are greatly indebted to Dan Lebenta for access to his unpublished review paper "Timeout from Positive Reinforcement," upon which we drew heavily in the preparation of this chapter.

Brown, 1967; Zeilberger et al., 1968), improper eating habits (Barton et al., 1970; Herrickson and Doughty, 1967), thumb-sucking (Baer, 1962), and inappropriate speech (Barton, 1970; McReynolds, 1969).

Timeout is a popular modification technique because under some circumstances it can produce immediate suppression of the unwanted response (McMillan, 1967), and is extremely effective in suppressing behavior if an alternative response is available that produces the same density of reinforcement but without timeout (Holz, Azrin and Ayllon, 1963). For example, if a child's cooperative play with his siblings earns frequent reinforcement but his quarreling with them produces a timeout, the quarrel-contingent timeout can control his disruptive behavior. The child has a reinforced behavioral alternative available – cooperative play. It has also been found that punished responding is not resumed when timeout is removed if an alternative response is provided (Holz, Azrin, and Ayllon, 1963). Thus, the availability of alternative responses increases the durability of timeout (TO) effects.

There is also some evidence that with animal subjects, at least, *brief* TO's (40 seconds) produced as much response suppression as did electric shocks. However, unlike the shock punishment, TO produced no generalized suppression of responding, nor did the subjects adapt to the TO causing it to lose its effectiveness (McMillan, 1967). The research evidence supports the conclusion that response-contingent timeout can be a highly effective suppression technique.

Implementation. The use of the term "timeout" implies that the modification agent has identified and is withholding the positive reinforcer maintaining the target behavior. In practice, however, it is sometimes difficult to identify the reinforcer. Isolating the child to achieve timeout sometimes allows one to implement the technique without having pinpointed the relevant reinforcing stimulus. Because isolation withdraws so many potential sources of reinforcement (e.g., interaction with others, accessibility of foods or interesting activities), it is very likely that isolation, in fact, produces a timeout from access to positive reinforcement. There are exceptions, however, when attempts to use isolation timeout have failed because of failure to identify the maintaining reinforcers (Risley, 1968). Failures in the use of timeout may be especially likely to occur when the undesirable behavior can be engaged in while the child is in isolation, as is the case for self-stimulation, which sometimes appears to be intrinsically reinforcing.

Timeout location. One must use discretion in selecting an isolation location. A lively, crowded school hallway may provide rich sources of reinforcement for the child who is supposedly timed out from classroom activities. The child's own bedroom may contain attractive toys, books, a television set, or other amusements that preclude its use as a timeout room.

For these reasons, bathrooms are often used as isolation areas; in the home, corridors and stairways may be convenient locations. In classroom settings, younger children might be seated in a chair facing the wall, and older children could be sent to vacant school rooms. In individual tutoring projects, the tutor can turn away and busy himself with other activities or can leave the tutoring room in order to administer a timeout to a child. For a very young child, the adult can simply turn away from the child briefly to give him a timeout.

Beware of using highly unpleasant locations for timeout rooms. Dark and cobwebbed basement rooms or stifling closets can frighten the child severely and cause him to engage in much emotional and escape behavior. The object is to deter, not to frighten the child.

Timeout duration. As yet no firm guidelines are available for selection of a TO duration. In research and clinical reports, TO's have varied in length from as brief as a few seconds to as long as several hours (Johnston, 1972). Most clinical programs directed toward children have employed TO durations of between 30 seconds and ten minutes. Generally, the younger the child, the briefer the TO used. The decision is usually made on empirical grounds with the contingency manager imposing the briefest TO that still remains effective. Brevity is desirable for several reasons: first, it minimizes the time during which the child is removed from the learning situation. Second, very long TO's have been found to disrupt *both* correct and incorrect responding of animal subjects (Ferster and Appel, 1961; Zimmerman and Bayden, 1963; Zimmerman and Ferster, 1963). That is, extremely long TO's* can have a generally suppressing effect on behavior.

Since the TO situation is itself aversive, any behaviors the child engages in during timeout are necessarily paired with aversive stimuli. Should he begin to behave very acceptably, and should the TO duration be very long, such as an hour, it is possible for his good behavior to be associated with continuing aversive stimulation. In effect, he would be punished while behaving desirably, an unfortunate circumstance. The longer the TO period, the greater is the probability that the child will behave quietly and constructively, performances that are necessarily paired with aversive stimuli (Johnston, 1972).

Moreover, long timeouts should be avoided for humanitarian reasons (White, Nielsen, and Johnson, 1972). We consider it ethically undesirable to subject people (especially children) to unpleasant experiences that are of excessive length or intensity. The experience should be just aversive enough to

*TO's are long or short in relative terms and depending upon subject species. In work with pigeons, Ferster and Appel (1961) refer to a 120-second TO duration as long, but 120 seconds would not be considered a long TO to administer human subjects.

suppress the deviant behavior, but no more so.

Brief timeout periods can prove effective when the child has not previously been exposed to longer timeout intervals. White, Nielsen, and Johnson (1972) have found that a one-minute timeout period in isolation reduced retarded children's aggressive and self-injurious behaviors, but only when the one-minute timeout preceded rather than followed the child's experiencing longer (15 and 30-minute) timeout punishments. When the longer timeouts were applied first, subsequent use of the brief timeout was counterproductive. It seems, then, that it is advisable to begin treatment with quite brief timeout durations and then increase the duration should that prove necessary.

In any case, use a timer. A kitchen timer is inexpensive and handy for this purpose. Set the timer for the interval you had previously decided to use, then keep the child in TO until that interval has elapsed. Failure to use a timer can easily result in your forgetting to release the child from TO. We have little idea of the effects of the resulting undeservedly long TO's, but they can be most disconcerting for both child and manager.

In some instances the child himself can determine the length of his TO. Many teachers and clinicians instruct children who are misbehaving to stay in isolation until they feel they can behave themselves. The child then makes the decision himself regarding when he will return from TO. Whether this procedure is effective must be determined individually on a trial-and-error basis. One possible difficulty is that the child can keep the TO duration so brief that its aversive properties are minimal. In such a situation, the aversiveness of TO may be outweighed by the caretaker attention involved in scolding the child and instructing him to take a TO. If you are aware of these possible problems beforehand, you are forearmed when the situation actually arises.

Return from TO. It is important not to terminate TO because of a child's protests against it or his assaults on the timeout room. Your giving way in the face of such behavior may well act to reinforce the child's violence. Clear the timeout room of delicate and valuable items in advance. If the child throws water around the room or otherwise messes things up, have him clean up before he is released from timeout, and make extra minutes in timeout contingent upon room damage.

How to administer TO. Escort the child to the room in a calm but firm and businesslike manner. Tell him the rules for the length of time he must stay in TO and under what conditions he can earn release. Do not argue; just give instructions, then carry out those rules. Use a timer to make sure that you do.

After you have confined the child to a timeout room, don't hover around outside the door to issue continuing instructions. This will usually only prolong his protests.

It is advisable to allow the child's return from TO only when his misbehavior has ceased for some predetermined interval. If he has been timed out for tantrums, for example, you may want to require a five-minute timeout plus at least ten consecutive seconds of silence (no tantrums) as a condition for return from TO. Allowing a child to return while he is still yelling or kicking can reinforce that type of behavior, whereas terminating the TO contingent upon good behavior will reinforce the desired behavior, such as ceasing tantrums and other protest behavior (Bostow and Bailey, 1969; Hawkins, Peterson, Schweid, and Bijou, 1966; Wolf, Risley, Johnston, Harris, and Allen, 1967; Wolf et al., 1964; Zeilberger et al., 1968). As Johnston (1972) has pointed out in his review of the effects of punishment on human behavior, various criteria have been used for scheduling release from TO, for example: (a) when the punished response terminates, or (b) after the end of some undesirable behavior plus some predetermined additional time interval, or (c) following the occurrence of some appropriate response. One possible problem with the use of the last-named criterion for release from TO is that the TO may lose its aversive properties for the child who learns that he can be released nearly immediately from TO should he quickly begin behaving appropriately. He is then free to return immediately to the original situation, having experienced a very mild and probably ineffective punishment. Table 6-2 presents the preliminary decisions you must make before using TO.

Table 6-2 Preliminary Decisions in the Use of TO

Before using TO:

1. Decide upon the TO contingency – for example, that each time the child destroys a toy he will immediately be given a TO.
2. Decide upon the method of delivering the TO. You might, for instance, decide to isolate the child in a bathroom or bedroom, you might place him in a chair and turn it toward a wall, or you might briefly extinguish the lights in a classroom or playroom. If you have been feeding the child and wish to TO some behavior that occurs at mealtimes, you might briefly take away the child's plate.
3. Decide upon the length of the TO.
4. Choose a pre-TO warning if you wish to use one.
5. Make rules concerning the conditions under which the child is to be returned or released from TO.

Example of TO. As an example of a TO procedure, a parent might use TO to decrease a young child's rate of pinching people and pets. He first explains the procedure to the child – "You shouldn't pinch. Whenever you pinch anyone or pinch the dog, you will have to stay in your room." Then, upon the next pinching incident, the parent says, "Timeout for pinching," and escorts the child quickly and firmly to the bedroom and closes the door for the predetermined interval – say five minutes. The first time TO is used, the child may protest loudly, try to open his door, argue, knock on the door, and perhaps cry for a longer time than the scheduled five minutes of TO. Since the parent will not wish to reinforce any of these protest actions, he tells the child that he (the child) will be released when he stops crying and calms down. This instruction is given only once in order to minimize the length of the protest and to minimize the possibility of reinforcing arguing. As a result, the child's anger outbursts in response to TO will rapidly diminish after the first several TO's are administered.

Pre-TO stimuli. A stimulus associated with and discriminative for TO can acquire conditioned punishing properties. These properties can include behavior suppression; thus, for some instances TO need not be administered. The presentation of the pre-TO stimulus will suffice to suppress the target behavior.* The pre-TO stimulus presented a child can consist of a verbal warning ("Stop that, or you'll have a timeout"), a warning look, or a gesture. Since a verbal warning frequently generates an argument over whether a TO is merited, some nonverbal stimulus is desirable. A hand signal is easy to use, requires no special equipment, and only requires that the manager attract the child's attention. We have found it helpful to use the hand signal used by basketball referees to warn players of the imminence of a technical foul assessment.** This gesture consists of placing one hand at a right angle to the other in a "T" arrangement. Referees find it most effective.

When to use TO. TO will act as a suppressor when the child's behavior is maintained on a relatively rich reinforcement schedule. If, instead, the child is on a lean intermittent schedule, he may actually choose TO over some schedules of positive reinforcement, during which his chances of being reinforced are remote in any case (Appel, 1963; Azrin, 1961; Thompson, 1964)

*In animal laboratory experiments, however, Leitenberg (1965) has found that stimuli preceding TO from positive reinforcement have an accelerating rather than a decelerating effect on response rate. This acceleration effect does not seem to occur in applied work with children, so don't worry about it; just be alert and be guided by the demonstrable impact your procedures have on your child-client's behavior.

**Our thanks to Sid Gelfand for suggesting the use of this signal. His thousands of hours spent watching basketball on television appear not entirely wasted.

Of course, he can "choose" TO by simply misbehaving while a TO contingency is in effect. As always, you, as well as the child, are controlled by the program you have devised for him. If your TO procedure does not seem to be working, it is possible that the child is not receiving enough positive reinforcement for his desirable behavior. Surprisingly, TO may also be less effective when reinforcement frequency is very high (Thomas, 1964), so the subject has relatively little to lose since reinforcers are readily obtainable.

Undesirable effects. TO can stimulate emotional behavior such as crying, screaming, and physical attacks, particularly if the TO recipient must be physically removed to an isolation chamber (Ferster and Skinner, 1957). TO may be difficult to administer when the "child" is a large, protesting adolescent and the procedure calls for isolating him against his will. The contingency manager must then be prepared for attacks directed against property in the timeout room and possibly against himself.

Advantages of TO. One of the practical advantages of the use of TO is that it can be administered relatively unemotionally. It is therefore not as upsetting or emotionally arousing to both manager and child as is corporal or verbal punishment. Child and manager are separated from each other in TO, so that they do not have the opportunity to further taunt or threaten each other as they can when physical or verbal punishment is in progress. The separation period gives each participant a chance to calm down and to approach the situation more objectively. Consequently, interpersonal friction tends to be briefer and less violent when TO is used. In fact, in a carefully controlled experiment, Wahler (1969) found that TO not only reduced children's oppositional behavior, but also apparently increased the reinforcement power of parents' social attention toward their children.

A second advantage previously mentioned is that TO periods can be relatively brief and still effective. TO's of less than one minute may suffice in work with preschool children. This means that not much learning time is lost in attempts at misbehavior suppression. In view of these desirable features, TO is certainly a suppression procedure worthy of your consideration.

Probe Questions for Part 2, Chapter 6

1. Why is it not a good idea to use physical punishment to attempt to reduce a child's fighting and quarreling?

2. State the potential problems associated with the use of punishment.

3. If you do decide to use a punishment procedure, what guidelines should you follow to insure its effectiveness?

4. Discuss the advantages and disadvantages in the use of TO.

5. What precautions should a therapist take in employing a timeout procedure?

6. Suppose that a child whom you have put into his bedroom for a timeout period begins beating on his door with a hammer. What would you do and why?

Behavioral Objectives for Part 3, Chapter 6

Study of this section should enable you to:

1. Describe a response-cost contingency, the conditions governing its effectiveness, and its merits relative to physical punishment and timeout.

2. Describe stimulus satiation, restraint, and stimulus change, and the situations in which each might be an effective modification strategy.

Part 3. Response Cost, Stimulus Satiation, Restraint, and Stimulus Change

RESPONSE COST

Another punishment procedure that is seeing increased clinical use is response cost. The response-cost procedure most commonly used consists of allowing the individual to accumulate, but not consume, a supply of reinforcers, some of which can be confiscated following misbehavior (Kazdin, 1972; Weiner, 1962). In effect, the child is fined for violating the rules. Since it is relatively difficult to arrange for the removal of primary reinforcers, conditioned reinforcers such as points, tokens, or money are usually removed contingent upon the child's making an incorrect response. This most often takes place in a situation in which the child is also earning these same conditioned reinforcers for his desirable performances (see Part 2, Chapter 5). As an illustration, a parent might set up a home program whereby his child earns set amounts of money for performing various household chores, but also loses money for specified misbehaviors such as fighting with siblings or failing to return home on time. Response-cost procedures are also frequently used in token economy programs (Atthowe and Krasner, 1968; Phillips, Phillips, Fixsen, and Wolf, 1971) and are sometimes incorporated into individual contingency contacts (Stuart, 1971).

Deprivation of privileges following misbehavior also constitutes a response-cost procedure. A teacher might deprive a child of recess time for making excessive noise during class, or a parent might deprive a child of television viewing time and of his dessert in an effort to control his child's lying or stealing. In the preceding examples, tokens or points are neither administered nor confiscated, although the child pays a penalty for improper behavior. While these techniques are employed frequently by parents and teachers, we have as yet little research evidence regarding their proper use or effectiveness (Kazdin, 1972). Consequently, we recommend that you make use of token reinforcers and withdraw them and withhold the back-up reinforcer contingent upon the child's behavioral deviancy.

Effectiveness. Laboratory research indicates that response cost can suppress behavior more effectively than some TO procedures (Weiner, 1962). Weiner found that response suppression was immediate and almost complete with some subjects. The various clinical reports available also attest to response-cost effectiveness. It is notable that response cost does not typically produce the amount and intensity of emotional behavior characteristically associated with other punishment procedures.

Undesirable effects. Although most investigations of the effects of response-cost procedures have not revealed undesirable side effects (Kazdin, 1972; Leitenberg, 1965), two studies have reported anecdotal evidence of associated problems. Boren and Colman (1970) found that in a token reinforcement program for institutionalized delinquent soldiers, imposing fines for absenteeism at ward meetings resulted in greater absenteeism and rebellious behavior. Similarly, Meichenbaum, Bowers, and Ross (1968) reported that a response-cost contingency in a classroom token reinforcement program produced a decrease in the appropriate academic behavior of adolescent delinquent girls. The girls also protested the use of fines. In this latter study, however, the introduction of the fine contingency was accompanied by a reduction in the amount of money the girls could earn each day, so it is difficult to interpret the results unequivocally.

It may be that these adolescent and adult offenders had become so proficient in controlling others through threats and coercive techniques that they effectively deterred therapists from attempting treatment programs based on anything except positive reinforcement procedures. As Boren and Colman (1970, p. 32) commented, their delinquent soldiers were "strong and aggressive young men who could physically damage staff members . . . these patients reportedly had past histories of destructive behavior in response to aversive control."

In contrast, in work with younger, predelinquent boys, Phillips, Fixsen, and Wolf and their colleagues have found response-cost procedures to be a very effective ingredient of token reinforcement treatment programs (Phillips, 1968; Phillips et al., 1971; Wolf, Phillips, and Fixsen, 1972). Perhaps the age of the therapeutic subjects and the length of their history of antisocial, oppositional behavior are important considerations in the selection of appropriate modification techniques.

Requirements. In order to put a response-cost contingency into effect, you must create a situation in which:

1. Some level of positive reinforcement is administered to the child (so that you will have something to withdraw if necessary).

2. You have established the value of and are using conditioned reinforcers such as tokens, points, or money (Azrin and Holz, 1966).

If these two prerequisites are met, you can institute a response-cost procedure.

Implementation. After you have met the preceding requirements, decide the precise cost to be attached to each instance and type of misbehavior. Do not decide costs on the spur of the moment just as the child is misbehaving. Under such circumstances you are likely to be very angry and to overcharge the child. If the costs become too high and the reinforcement rate too low, he will naturally stop working. This may occur when the child has incurred so many fines that he must work hard to get out of debt. Decide the charges to be assessed at some other time and place, when you can make a more objective analysis. Unfortunately, we have no research evidence on the optimal earnings-to-fines ratios. You must simply be alert to the child's behavioral responsiveness to your program and be ready to readjust his pay and fine values when necessary. Normally, this will involve some negotiation with the child himself.

Beware of relying too heavily on fines. It is often easier to think of how to fine a child than of how to shape a desired competing behavior. Be very sparing in the fines assessed or the whole learning situation will become aversive for the child and he will attempt to escape it. The police and courts make heavy use of fines – consider how popular they are.

Example

Phillips (1968) and his colleagues have used token reinforcement and response-cost (fines) procedures to modify the behavior of juvenile offenders in a home-style rehabilitation agency. The token reinforcers were points that could be exchanged once a week for a variety of back-up reinforcers such as spending money, snacks, free time, and the use of a television set, a bicycle, tools, or game equipment. Each boy carried his own index card on which his points were entered as he earned them and point deductions were made for his transgressions. Table 6-3 shows some of the target behaviors and their point-worth as used by Phillips.

Table 6-3 Prices, Costs, and Earning Possibilities Used in the Achievement Place Program

	Behaviors that Earned Points	*Points*
1)	Watching news on TV or reading the newspaper	300 per day
2)	Cleaning and maintaining neatness in one's room	500 per day
3)	Keeping one's person neat and clean	500 per day
4)	Reading books	5 to 10 per page
5)	Aiding house-parents in various household tasks	20 to 1000 per task
6)	Doing dishes	500 to 1000 per meal
7)	Being well dressed for an evening meal	100 to 500 per meal

8)	Performing homework	500 per day
9)	Obtaining desirable grades on school report cards	500 to 1000 per grade
10)	Turning out lights when not in use	25 per light
	Behaviors that Lost Points	*Points*
1)	Failing grades on the report card	500 to 1000 per grade
2)	Speaking aggressively	20 to 50 per response
3)	Forgetting to wash hands before meals	100 to 300 per meal
4)	Arguing	300 per response
5)	Disobeying	100 to 1000 per response
6)	Being late	10 per minute
7)	Displaying poor manners	50 to 100 per response
8)	Engaging in poor posture	50 to 100 per response
9)	Using poor grammar	20 to 50 per response
10)	Stealing, lying, or cheating	10,000 per response
	Privileges that Cost Points	*Points*
1)	Bicycle use	1000 per week
2)	TV viewing time	1000 per week
3)	Permission to go downtown	1000 per week
4)	Permission to stay up past bedtime	1000 per week
5)	Permission to come home late from school	1000 per week
6)	Snacks	1000 per week
7)	Allowance	1000 per week
8)	Games	500 per week
9)	Access to tools	500 per week

Note: From Phillips (1968).

This token economy was adjusted so that a boy who completed all of his assigned tasks and who had incurred minimal fines could obtain all the back-up reinforcer privileges available without his having to do extra work. The results available thus far indicate that this type of program has considerable promise for treating delinquent boys (Phillips, 1968; Phillips et al., 1971).

Stimulus Satiation

Satiation methods provide another method of response suppression. The procedure consists of providing the subject with reinforcers so frequently and in such quantities that he becomes completely sated. The stimuli that previously served as reinforcers then become neutral or aversive stimuli for him, and he rejects them. At the same time, the responses formerly maintained by these stimuli are weakened.

In cases in which the reinforcing event involves a particular action on the child's part (such as lighting matches or tearing up magazines), the repetition of the action may result in fatigue or boredom (Welsh, 1971). The association of the previously preferred activity with these negative emotional states can confer conditioned aversive properties upon the activity and lead the child to avoid it.

This method is rarely used for a variety of practical reasons. Satiation procedures are impractical when the reinforcing stimuli are not available in sufficiently large supply or when they are too expensive or are potentially harmful when administered in large quantities. Satiation, then, is a technique best used in cases in which the particular reinforcer involved is inappropriate for use by the child. It may be inappropriate because its use exposes the child to ridicule. For example, a four-year-old child who sucks a pacifier might well be the object of scorn and might profit from satiation treatment. Satiation would consist of requiring him to keep the pacifier in his mouth for long periods each day. Or the reinforcer may be inappropriate because it is inconvenient or irritating to others – as in the case of hoarding. The child who hoards the family's supply of facial tissue, soap, light bulbs, snacks, or towels is a case in point.

Implementation. The suggestions offered here are based upon the work of Ayllon (1963), who used satiation techniques to cure a hospitalized psychotic woman of towel hoarding – a behavior pattern that annoyed and inconvenienced the nursing staff.

To implement a satiation procedure, you should:

1. Remove any measures that may have been in effect to attempt to restrict the child's access to the reinforcer. If the stimulus item has been hidden, you may place it out in full view; if you have been confiscating it,

stop.

2. Offer the item frequently and repeatedly to the child. You may have to follow this procedure for a matter of days or weeks. Ayllon (1963) presented his towel hoarder with up to 60 towels a day for a period of three weeks.

3. Continue to supply the item to the child until he rejects it. It would be safest to continue until you encounter emphatic and repeated rejection of the former reinforcer. Good evidence of the time to stop is that the child avoids or attempts to escape from the stimulus.

Welsh (1971) has reported using stimulus satiation techniques to eliminate inappropriate fire-setting in two seven-year-old boys. Since these were not controlled studies, however, one cannot very confidently assert that the observed behavior change resulted from the treatment manipulations. The situation is further complicated by the fact that the therapist not only required each boy to continue to light matches over several satiation sessions, but also taught them how to light matches and to burn them safely – an alternative behavior. Nevertheless, the procedure merits examination.

Each boy was brought into the therapy room and was provided 20 boxes of small wooden matches. He was told that he would be learning how to light matches properly, and was instructed to light only one match at a time, to close the box cover before striking a match, and to hold the match over the ashtray at all times. Satiation sessions were approximately 50 minutes long and consisted of the boys' lighting match after match according to the therapist's instructions.

During the third satiation session, one boy requested to be allowed to play with the other toys in the therapy room but was forced to sit at the table and light ten matches. Then he was allowed to play with toys of his choice for the remainder of the session. Welsh reports that the fire-setting behavior had not returned at the time of follow-up observation six months later. A second boy required four satiation sessions and was also reported to have refrained from fire-setting in a six-month interval following treatment. Despite the apparent success of this technique, beginning student therapists should not attempt to treat so potentially dangerous a problem as fire-setting (see the Chapter 2 guidelines for choice of a problem behavior).

Limitations. It is possible to recover from satiation. The thrice daily cycle of eating until full, then pausing until the next meal, is a familiar example of satiation and recovery. In this case recovery is relatively rapid. In treatment applications it may be necessary to repeat the satiation process more than once in order to achieve lasting effects. Indeed, it may not work at all with some reinforcers. Very little clinical evidence is yet available to provide us with the information necessary to decide under what circumstances satiation will be effective.

In addition, satiation may prove physically dangerous in some cases. Certainly you can't use candy satiation with a diabetic child, and you may even not wish to use it with a child with tooth-decay problems. Be sure the satiation procedure represents no danger to the child (and, of course, that no one else is trying to deny the child access to the reinforcer at the same time and in the same situation in which you are attempting stimulus satiation).

Unlike punishment procedures, suppression is not immediate with satiation. If the behavior must be eliminated immediately, satiation is not the procedure of choice.

In summary, there is some, but little, information that satiation can be an effective response-suppression procedure for clinical use when the reinforcer in question is inappropriate for the child. Its effects are not always permanent, however, and it does not produce immediate suppression. If immediacy and permanence are required, it would be better to use some punishment technique.

Restraint

Sometimes it is easier to change the environment so that a response cannot occur than it is to teach the child not to perform that particular response. We sometimes see parents tie mittens on their baby's hands to prevent or restrain him from sucking his thumb. Or they may place him in a playpen to restrict him from contact with dangerous or fragile household objects. Restraint procedures are used most frequently with infants, less so with older children. Restraint is often used in cases in which it is thought useless or not worthwhile to teach the child to restrict his own behavior and with children who are not agile or clever enough to circumvent the restraints.

Limitations. The greatest problem associated with the use of restraint procedures is that they are designed only to physically prevent the occurrence of an ordinarily reinforced behavior. No new behavior patterns are taught, so the target behavior resumes as soon as the restraint is removed. Consequently, while restraint procedures can totally prevent some misbehaving from occurring, they usually do not have an enduring effect on behavior (Holz and Azrin, 1963).

Teaching competing behaviors. It is, of course, possible to teach the child a competing behavior while using restraint to prevent misbehavior. An example would be a young child who attempts to grab a toy from another child. You might physically restrain him from doing so, while at the same time instructing him to share. Instruct him that he will be rewarded (e.g., given a chance to play with the desired toy) if, and only if, he completes some required interval of cooperative play. One potential drawback is that such a restraint procedure may actually prove appealing to the culprit, since it involves parental attention and physical contact, both of which may have reinforcing properties for most children.

Example

Foxx and Azrin (1973) have successfully used a technique they term "overcorrection" to control self-stimulatory behavior in retarded and autistic children. The overcorrection procedure combines elements of verbal reprimand (saying "No" to the child), physical restraint (holding the child's jaw, head, or arms to prevent self-stimulatory mouthing, head-weaving, and hand-clapping, respectively), and practice of an acceptable behavior incompatible with self-stimulation. For example, the corrective behavior introduced for mouthing objects was cleaning the child's mouth with antiseptic mouthwash; the corrective behavior for head-weaving was the child's holding her head up, down, or straight; and the corrective behavior for hand-clapping was the child's holding his hands in one of five positions: above his head, directly in front of him, clasped together, behind his back, or thrust into his pockets. The therapist's physical restraints were faded gradually from forceful holding, to touching, to shadowing the child's head or hands with the therapist's hands, as the child's behavior came more under instructional control of the therapist's verbal warning to desist from self-stimulation. These training procedures were in effect weekdays from 9:00 a.m. to 3:00 p.m. in a day-care treatment program and were demonstrably superior to other control measures including (a) food and praise for refraining from self-stimulation, (b) a sharp slap on the thigh for self-stimulation, or (c) painting the child's hand with a foul-tasting solution to reduce mouthing. As in other programs that involve the use of restraint, the therapist must be physically present for a good deal of the time during which the child engages in the taboo behavior and must be close enough to the child to restrain him immediately after the inception of the behavior.

Be careful in the use of restraints. You may be inadvertently reinforcing misbehavior or training escape behavior. In any event, you are only temporarily suppressing the target response. Whenever feasible, try to promote a competing prosocial behavior when you use a restraint procedure.

Stimulus Change

You can temporarily suppress a response by removing the S^D's associated with that response and substituting new and different stimuli. Parents frequently use distraction tactics to prevent infants and toddlers from engaging in dangerous or prohibited activities. The parent simply changes the situation by calling the child's attention to another toy or activity. As an example of a different stimulus-change procedure, consider the case of an overweight child who begins consuming snacks the moment the television set is turned on. Removing the television stimulus and replacing it with radio, phonograph, or reading might temporarily disrupt the child's eating pattern. Note, however, that if the same reinforcement contingency remains in effect after the stimulus change, the target-response rate will probably recover (Azrin and Holz, 1966). But the momentary response suppression associated with stimulus change may suffice to allow the shaping of a desirable response alternative. Since the stimulus change effect, when it does occur, is temporary, this procedure is rarely used alone in behavior modification practice.

Summary and Conclusions

We have now reviewed the various methods used to decrease the frequency of changeworthy behavior. In using any of these methods, you should make sure you are on firm ethical ground and that you are using the least harsh intervention consistent with the goal of effecting behavior change. In very few, if any, circumstances is it advisable to use a response-reduction tactic alone rather than in combination with some shaping procedure or reinforcement of preexisting prosocial behavior. In fact, in many circumstances the most desirable way of reducing a changeworthy behavior is to place it on extinction and to reinforce an incompatible positive response. Now that you have read descriptions of the various means of modifying excess behavior, review Table 6-1 and make a final determination of the method you will employ.

Probe Questions for Part 3, Chapter 6

1. What is response cost, and how is this procedure usually employed in everyday life?

2. Describe the behavioral problems for which response cost would, and those for which it would not, be an appropriate treatment.

3. Why is satiation used less often than other response-reduction techniques?

4. Give examples of situations in which it is desirable to use restraint procedures. When is restraint inappropriate?

5. How would you use an overcorrection procedure to control a child's fingernail-biting ?

Behavioral Objectives for Part 1, Chapter 7

After studying Part 1 of this chapter, you should be able to state why:

1. It is important to obtain reliable data.

2. It is necessary to determine the reliability of your data during each phase of your study.

3. Your child-client should be informed of the reasons for the presence of an observer.

4. The data sheets from coobservers should be compared immediately after each reliability check.

Finally, you should be able to:

5. State the three questions that require answering *before* you determine the reliability of your data.

CHAPTER 7

Reliability

Part 1. Introduction and Preliminaries

INTRODUCTION

The technical meaning of reliability is not unlike the colloquial meaning. If a friend or acquaintance is unreliable, he is inconsistent, and hence little confidence can be placed in him. So it is with data. Behavioral data are reliable to the degree that measurements from independent observers are consistent or in agreement.* Consequently, when you assess the reliability of data obtained from human observers, you must compare data from at least two *independent* observers who have made simultaneous observations of samples of behavior.

Attainment of a high degree of observer reliability is a crucial requirement for your study. If your data are highly reliable, you will be able to detect small as well as large changes produced in the target behavior. The absence of change then can be attributed to inadequate treatment procedures and not to faulty measurement techniques. On the other hand, if your data

*This is a restrictive definition of reliability. In other kinds of experiments reliability may involve the consistency of subjects' performances over time, situations, etc. (See Anastasi, 1968.)

have poor or unknown reliability, you may be unable to detect or demonstrate change no matter how dramatic the change actually might be. Failure to check the reliability of your data may result in data of questionable accuracy, which consequently would be meaningless.

In this chapter we will describe the steps you should follow in comparing the data from two independent observers. We will also introduce the distinction between the reliability of a session score and the reliability of smaller unit scores, such as trial scores within sessions. We will discuss the concept of observer bias and drift, and then describe for you the data gathering requirements and calculation formulas for quantifying these concepts.

COLLECTING DATA

Before you begin to collect formal baseline data, check the reliability of your observations. Recruit a second observer (or your partner) and repeat the reliability assessment procedures described in Chapter 2, but using the new response definitions and observation tactics. You will also want to include a reliability probe (i.e., another reliability check) at each successive phase of your project to insure that you are not altering definitions or in some other way deteriorating as a data gathering instrument, a danger discussed at some length in Part 3 of this chapter.

Before you begin data collection, see that both you and your fellow observer are completely familiar with the behavior definitions, the data sheet, and the use of any timing devices you might need. A brief "dress rehearsal" quickly exposes improper preparation.

If the observations are to be carried out in some quasi-private place, such as in a home or unused classroom, be certain that your fellow observer and the child have been introduced to one another. Needless to say, the unexpected appearance of even familiar persons can be disruptive, so provide your child-client with some understanding of the reason for the observer's presence.

While collecting data, position yourself and the reliability checker in such a way that you will both have an unimpeded view of the child. However, be certain that you are not so close together that you cannot collect the data independently. Interobserver reliability estimates are meaningless if one observer copies or is in some way influenced by the other observer's recordings. Ideally, you should not even be able to tell whether the other observer is writing anything down at any given time. If you are using wrist counters, the observers should not be able to hear the click of one another's counters.

Check one another's data sheets *immediately after* the observation period, while behavior incidents are still fresh in your mind. If disagreements occur, as they probably will, develop rules to resolve questionable incidents. For example, assume that tantruming was the target behavior and duration data were being collected. One of the observers might click off his stopwatch when the child stopped kicking his mother's shins; the other observer might not click off his stopwatch until the child stopped both kicking and throwing tableware at his mother. A decision should then be made as to which criterion will be used.

More frequently, disagreements arise when a general class of behavior is being observed, such as appropriate classroom behavior, and the observers do not have an exhaustive list of what constitutes the general class. When a behavior not previously considered occurs, the observers might then disagree concerning its classification. If this happens, the observers should decide how the behavior will be classfied when it again occurs, and should add that behavior to the appropriate list so that future occurrences will be reliably categorized.

PRELIMINARY CONSIDERATIONS

Assume that you and your reliability checker have obtained data in a format similar to that given in Table 7-1 below. Depending upon which of the

Table 7-1 Example of a Two (Number of Observers) by K (Number of Intervals) Table for Interobserver Trial Reliability Data

	1	2	3	4	5	6	7	...	k
Observer 1									
Observer 2									

three types of data acquisition systems you employed, the number of recording or observation intervals will vary from a minimum of eight (if you used the tally or duration method) to some number much larger than that (if you used the interval method). The numerical values you obtain for these recording intervals will also vary depending upon which data acquisition method you used. For tally or duration data, each recording interval will be scored either zero or some positive number, indicating the frequency or duration of the behavior. For interval data, each recording interval will be scored either zero (the behavior did not occur in that interval) or one (the behavior did occur in that interval).

In order to assess the reliability of your data, you first make three basic decisions (Johnson and Bolstad, 1973, pp. 10-17).

1. The first decision requires specification of the *score unit* on which reliability will be assessed. If your target behavior is a single response, such as the number of diapers soiled or the amount of time spent watching TV, the score units checked for reliability are simply the numbers noted in the recording intervals on your data sheets.

The problem is more complicated, however, if the target behavior is really a *response class* or category that includes a number of component behaviors. Consider the target response "physical aggression toward peers," which includes four component responses – hitting, kicking, scratching, and shoving. If data had been collected on each of these four separate behaviors, reliability could be calculated on either the sum of hits, kicks, scratches, and shoves (the total physical aggression scores) in each recording interval, or on each of the four separate component scores in each recording interval. Which of the two reliabilities (total score or component scores) should be calculated depends on the score unit that will be used in graphing and data analysis. If total physical aggression is the primary dependent variable, then these scores should provide the basis of the reliability assessment. If, instead, each of the four "aggression" responses will be analyzed separately (for example, in a multiple baseline design), then each of the four scores should be examined separately for reliability.

2. The second decision requires specification of the *time span* over which scores will be summed for purposes of reliability assessment. Reliability could be caluculated on the scores in each of the eight or more recording intervals (see Table 7-1) for sessions in which two observers collected data. This is referred to as *trial* or interval reliability (Hartmann, 1974, c). Trial reliability primarily indicates the adequacy of behavior definitions and the thoroughness of observer training in the use of both these definitions and the observational equipment (such as coding sheets, recorders, and timers). Without a reasonable degree of interobserver reliability at the trial level, a study is

uninterpretable because of the ambiguous meaning of the basic data.

Reliability also could be calculated on the total session scores for each of the two observers. Referring again to Table 7-1, an observer's total session score is obtained by adding together his scores for the recording intervals within a session. A reliability analysis performed on these session totals is referred to as *session reliability.* Session reliability indicates how much confidence you can have in a session score. Put another way, it indicates the smallest difference between session scores that is not due to observer error.

Which of the two reliabilities (trial or session) is more appropriate for your study again depends on the scores used in graphing and data analysis. While session totals (or averages) are typically analyzed in applied behavioral studies, most behavior therapists (surprisingly) determine trial reliability alone. Because of its frequent use, the latter will receive the majority of our attention. An additional reason for our focus on trial reliability is that in most cases it provides a lower bound or minimum estimate of session reliability. Therefore, you can assume with reasonable assurance that if your trial reliability is acceptable, you session reliability will be as good or better.

3. The third and final decision concerns the *statistical method* used to summarize trial reliability data, a topic to which we will next direct our attention.

Probe Questions for Part 1, Chapter 7

1. Why is it important to obtain reliable data?

2. State how reliability might be improved by attention to simple human engineering factors.

3. How can the requirement of independence of data be violated in subtle ways during reliability probes?

4. Why might the positioning of observers during reliability probes affect the reliability of their ratings?

5. Distinguish between trial and session reliability. What scores are used in the determination of these two kinds of reliability?

Behavioral Objectives for Part 2, Chapter 7

After studying Part 2 of this chapter, you should be able to:

1. Summarize the data from a single session in a form that facilitates reliability computations.

2. Calculate the reliability of trial scores within a single session.

3. Overcome problems that contribute to poor reliability.

4. Determine whether your data are sufficiently reliable to begin your study.

Part 2. Trial Reliability

CALCULATING TRIAL RELIABILITY

There are two general approaches to determining trial reliability: percentage agreement indexes and reliability coefficients or correlations. We will discuss both percentage and correlational indexes of reliability and will tell you how to calculate both types of index for data collected by the interval, the tally, or the duration method. You should consult those sections that pertain particularly to the data collection method you are using.

Interval Recording

If you have used the interval method (occurrence-nonoccurrence), summarize your data by collapsing the two-by-k table (see Table 7-1 in Part 1 of this chapter) into a two-by-two table like the one shown in Table 7-2. This table will be used to summarize your observations – to indicate the number and kind of agreements and disagreements included in your observations.

Table 7-2 A Two-by-Two Table for Summarizing Interval Data

		Observer 2: 0	Observer 2: 1
Observer 1	1	A	B
Observer 1	0	C	D

Note: "0" indicates nonoccurrences and "1" indicates occurrences.

To collapse your data, follow these steps:

1. Count the number of observation intervals for which both observers agreed that the target behavior occurred. Enter this number in cell B.

2. Count the number of observation intervals for which both observers agreed that the target behavior did *not* occur. Enter this number in cell C.

3. Count the number of observation intervals for which Observer 1 indicated that the target behavior occurred while Observer 2 indicated that the target behavior did *not* occur. Enter this number in cell A.

4. Finally, count the number of observation intervals for which Observer 1 indicated that the target behavior did *not* occur while Observer 2 indicated that the target behavior did occur. Enter this number in cell D.

Consider the data given in Table 7-3.

Table 7-3 Example of a Small Set of Data Resulting from Interval Recording

	Recording Interval Number							
	1	2	3	4	5	6	7	8
Observer 1	0	1	1	1	0	0	0	1
Observer 2	0	1	1	0	1	0	1	1

The two-by-two summary table for these data is given in Table 7-4.

Be sure to check your entries in the summary table as follows: (1) Count the total frequencies included in the table; this number should be equal to the total number of intervals used on your data sheet. In the example above, these values should both be eight. (2) Compare the total number of "1's" and "0's" for each observer in the two-by-two table (see values given on the bottom and right margins) with the totals in the two-by-k table given on your data sheets. For example, the total frequency of "1's" marked by Observer 1 in the two-by-two table is obtained by summarizing the frequencies in the

Table 7-4 A Two-by-Two Summary Table of the Data Contained in Table 7-3

		Observer 2: 0	Observer 2: 3	
Observer 1	1	A: 1 (.13)	B: 3 (.37)	= 4 (.5)
	0	C: 2 (.25)	D: 2 (.25)	= 4 (.5)
		3 (.38)	5 (.62)	N = 8

Note: Proportions are given in parentheses.

first row of the two-by-two table; that is, A+B=4. Next, calculate one of the alternative measures of observer reliability.

Percentage agreement. Percentage agreement is obtained by adding the numbers in the agreement cells (cells B and C) and dividing by the sum of the number of agreements plus the number of disagreements (A+B+C+D); this value is then multiplied by 100.

$$\text{Percentage agreement} = [(B+C)/(A+B+C+D)] \times 100.$$

For example, for the two-by-two data given in Table 7-4, percentage agreement is 62.5% – i.e., $[(3+2)/(1+3+2+2)] \times 100 = 62.5\%$.

Percentage agreement is the measure of reliability most commonly used in current behavior modification work. While it is simply calculated and readily understood, it has certain undesirable characteristics, including overestimating the "true" reliability of the data.

Percentage agreement overestimates the reliability of data from a two-by-two, or any sized table by failing to correct for chance agreements. Consider, for example, the data given in Table 7-4. Based on the proportional values given in parentheses in this table, the proportion of agreements = .625. But how much of this agreement could be due to accidental or chance agreement?

The level of chance agreements for cell B is found by multiplying the two marginal proportions that intersect at cell B (i.e., .5 and .62). This Product = .31. Thus, .31/.37 or 84% of the agreement in cell B could be due to chance.

The chance agreements for cell C, the other agreement cell, are similarly found by multiplying the two marginal proportions that intersect at cell C (i.e., .5 and .38). This product = .19. Thus, .19/.25 or 76% of the agreements regarding nonoccurrences in cell C could be due to chance.

The sum of the expected agreements for cells B and C equals .50 (.31+.19). This value is the chance or expected agreement value for a two-by-two table with marginal proportions = .5, .5, .38, and .62. Thus, .50/.625 or 80% of the agreements in Table 7-4 could be due to chance.

Additional problems with percentage agreement as a summary reliability statistic have been discussed by Hartmann (1974, a, c).

Percentage effective agreement, the method described below, shares the advantages of percentage agreement, but provides a better estimate of the "true" reliability of the data.

Effective percentage agreement. Effective percentage agreement (Jensen, 1959) can be calculated in a straightforward manner from the data summarized in a two-by-two table on either occurrences or nonoccurrences of the target behavior. Effective percentage agreement for occurrences is sometimes used when the target behavior in an acceleration program has a very low rate of occurrence. In such cases, the C cell (agreement on nonoccurrences) is very large and "inflates" the usual percentage agreement index. Consequently, the C cell is excluded in the calculation of effective percentage agreement for occurrences.

Effective percentage agreement (for occurrences) = [B/(A+B+D)] x 100. For the data given in Table 7-4, this value = [3/(1+3+2)] x 100 = 50%.

Effective percentage of nonoccurrences, on the other hand, is sometimes used when the target behavior has a very high rate of occurrence – for example, during the beginning phases of a deceleration program. High rates of occurrence produce large values in the B cell (agreement on occurrences), which inflate the value of the percentage agreement statistic. Effective percentage agreement (for nonoccurrences) = [C/(A+C+D) x 100. Note that this formula excludes the B cell. For the data given in Table 7-4, effective percentage agreement for nonoccurrences = [2/(1+2+2)] x 100 = 40%.

Additional material on effective percentage agreement can be found in Hartmann (1974, c), Herbert (1973), and Jensen (1959).

Correlation coefficient. The correlation coefficient, in comparison to the percentage agreement methods already described, has superior statistical properties, but is somewhat more difficult to calculate. People not familar with correlational analysis find the correlational method more difficult to understand.

The calculation of the correlational measure of reliability (r_ϕ or the phi correlation for trial reliability with interval data) also begins with the data in a two-by-two summary table. Substitute the values from the summary table into the following formula:

$$r_\phi = \frac{BC - AD}{\sqrt{(A+B)(C+D)(A+C)(B+D)}}.$$

For example, with the data given in Table 7-4,

$$r_\phi = \frac{(3)(2) - (1)(2)}{\sqrt{(4)(4)(3)(5)}} = \frac{4}{15.49} = .26$$

Phi, like most other correlation coefficients, varies from -1.0 (complete disagreement) through .00 (chance agreement) through +1.0 (complete agreement). Unlike the previously described percentage agreement, phi does not overestimate the degree of agreement between observers.

> r_ϕ as described above for two-by-two table data provides nearly identical values to kappa, a reliability statistic for categorical data recently described by Cohen and others (Cohen, 1960, 1968; Fleiss, 1971, 1973; Krippendorff, 1970). Kappa is defined as (proportion of observed agreements – proportion of chance agreements)/(one –proportion of chance agreements). Kappa, unlike r_ϕ, can be applied to three-by-three and other larger square data tables. For example, kappa could be used to summarize the reliability of two or more behaviors simultaneously recorded using the interval technique in a multiple baseline design. The phi coefficient, if applied to these same data, would have to be calculated separately for each one of the two or more behaviors.

A sample work sheet for determining the interobserver reliability of trial data is presented in Table 7-5. After you have completed the calculations, enter the occurrence totals for Observer 1 and Observer 2 and the reliability measure on the appropriate lines of the Summary Table, Table 7-6.

Table 7-5 Sample Work Sheet for Trial Reliability Calculations when Using the Interval Recording Method

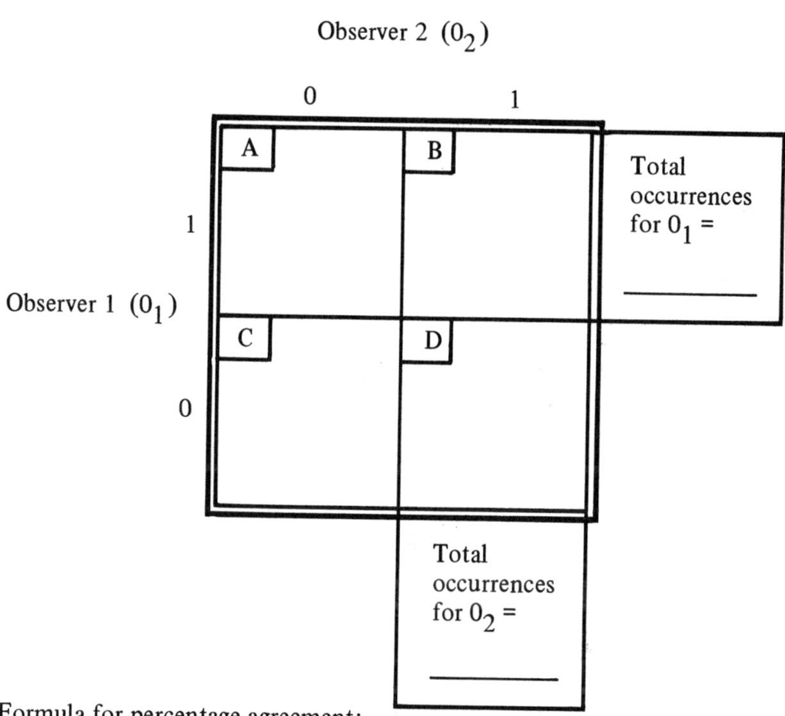

Formula for percentage agreement:

$[(B+C)/(A+B+C+D)] \times 100 =$

Formula for effective percentage agreement for:

Occurrences $[B/(A+B+D)] \times 100 =$

Non-occurrences $[C/(A+C+D)] \times 100 =$

Formula for r_ϕ:

$$(BC-AD) \Big/ \sqrt{(A+B)(C+D)(A+C)(B+D)} =$$

Table 7-6 Data Summary Sheet

Date	Time	Condition	Observer	Duration of Session or Number of Recording Interval	Raw Total	Adjusted Total	Reliability

Comments:

Note: For each session in which two observers collected data, bracket the two row entries in this table.

Examining Table 7-6 from left to right, the first four columns ask for simple information to identify the sessions. The next column entitled "duration of session or number of recording intervals" is included because occasionally you will have to deviate from your standard session length. With sessions variable in length, the scores must be adjusted in order to make all session scores comparable. The adjustment is based on the ratio of the length of the atypical session to the length of a standard session. For example, assume a standard observation session is 15-minutes long and contains 180 five-second intervals. If a session is shortened to 10 minutes, with 120 five-second intervals, the total for that session would have to be adjusted or prorated to make it comparable to other session totals. This adjusted total can be expressed as a percentage of the total intervals employed, in which case all totals should be expressed as percentages. Or the session total could be prorated. Proration of the 120 interval session total is accomplished by multiplying the obtained total by $\frac{180}{120}$ or 1.5 (See Chapter 10 for further discussion of this problem.) Whenever an adjustment technique is used, the adjusted total should be entered in the "adjusted total" column. The "comments" section at the bottom should be used to note information that will be used to qualify certain of the scores in your final report. For example, if a session has to be terminated immediately after its inception, the reason should be entered in the comments section and this fact noted on the final summary graph.

Tally or Duration Data

If you have used either the tally or duration method, you should have between eight and 12 pairs of scores resulting from your observations for purposes of reliability assessment. That is, the total observation period has been divided into eight to 12 discrete observation intervals, and each interval contains a score of zero or greater for each observer. If you have not divided your total observation interval into eight to 12 smaller intervals as we suggested in the previous chapter, your data may not be suitable for a correlational analysis. Hence, you may not be able to evaluate adequately the trial reliability on your frequency or duration data. If you slipped up this time, remedy the situation at the next opportunity.

Correlation coefficient. Although percentage agreement methods are sometimes used for tally or duration data, these methods are of questionable utility (see Hartmann, 1974, c; Herbert, 1973; Whelan, 1974). Consequently, you should calculate a correlational measure of reliability – in this case, the product-moment correlation ($r_{0_1 0_2}$). Although the formula looks forbidding, it is quite simple to calculate $r_{0_1 0_2}$, especially if you have access to a desk calculator.

$$r_{0_1 0_2} = \frac{N\Sigma 0_1 0_2 - \Sigma 0_1 \Sigma 0_2}{\sqrt{N\Sigma 0_1{}^2 - (\Sigma 0_1)^2}\ \sqrt{N\Sigma 0_2{}^2 - (\Sigma 0_2)^2}}$$

An example of the calculations required for the data given in Table 7-7 using this formula is shown in Table 7-8. A work sheet for calculating the product-moment correlation is given in Table 7-9.

Table 7-7 Sample Duration or Frequency Data

	Observation Intervals							
	1	2	3	4	5	6	7	8
Observer 1	5	0	17	0	0	8	7	1
Observer 2	4	1	17	0	0	6	9	0

For the small data tables with which you will be working, we have found that an easily calculated and acceptable estimate of $r_{0_1 0_2}$ can be obtained by calculating rho – the rank order correlation. The method of calculating rho can be found in most intermediate statistical texts.

After you have completed your calculations, triumphantly enter the value of $r_{0_1 0_2}$, as well as the session totals in the Data Summary Table, Table 7-6.

Calculation of session reliability. At the close of your project, after you have finished your last trial reliability probe and you have completed the Data Summary Table (Table 7-6), you can, if you wish, determine session reliability. To calculate session reliability, you use session totals – e.g., total performance frequency, duration, or occurrences for each session that was observed by two or more observers. These are the total scores you included in the "adjusted totals" column of the Data Summary Table. You should have eight to 12 of these sessions during which two observers collected data. Place the data from these eight to 12 sessions in the squares in Table 7-9 and perform the calculation for the product-moment correlations as directed in that table.

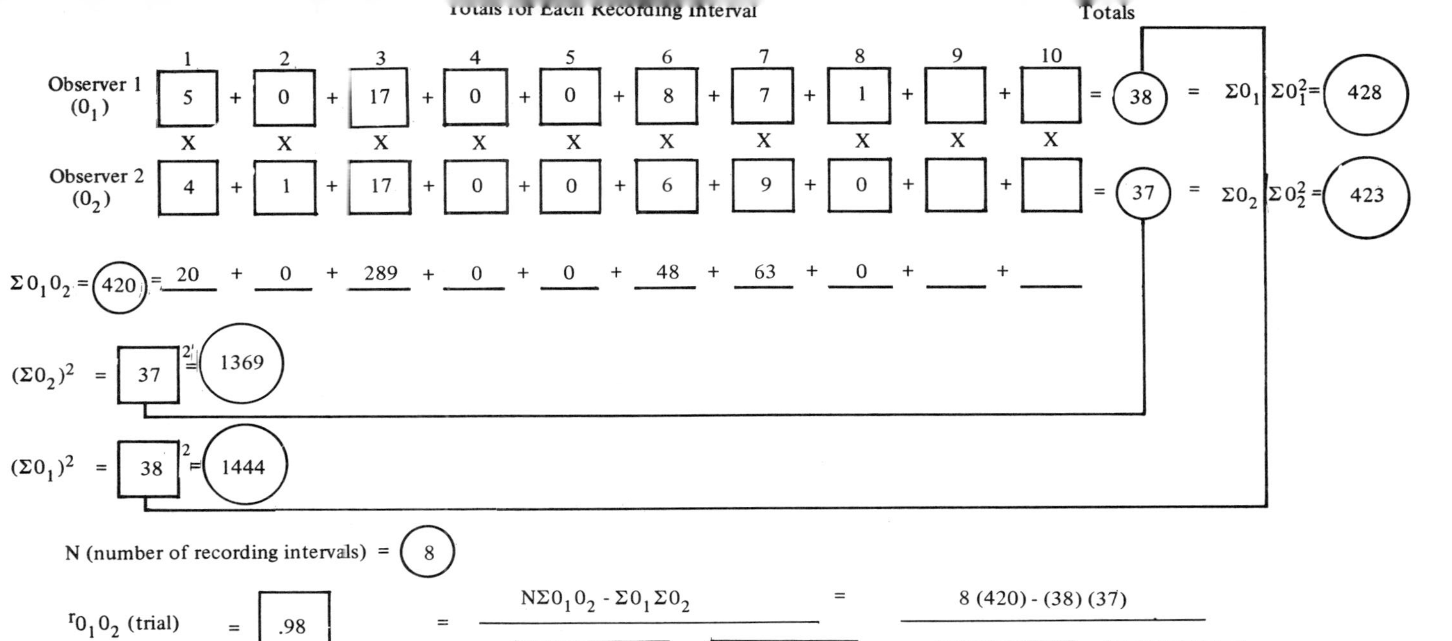

$$r_{0_1 0_2} = \frac{N\Sigma 0_1 0_2 - \Sigma 0_1 \Sigma 0_2}{\sqrt{N\Sigma 0_1{}^2 - (\Sigma 0_1)^2}\ \sqrt{N\Sigma 0_2{}^2 - (\Sigma 0_2)^2}} = \frac{8\,(420) - (38)\,(37)}{\sqrt{8\,(428) - 1444}\ \sqrt{8\,(423) - 1369}} = \frac{1954}{\sqrt{1980}\sqrt{2015}} = .98$$

Note: $\Sigma 0_1{}^2 = 5^2+0^2+17^2+0^2+0^2-8^2+7^2+1^2 = 428$

$\Sigma 0_2{}^2 = 4^2+1^2+17^2+0^2+0^2-6^2+9^2+0^2 = 423$

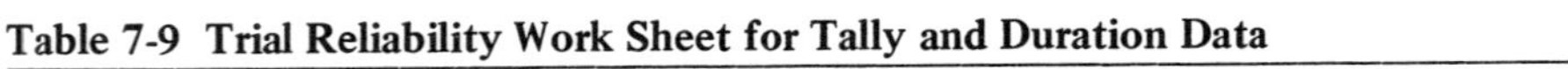

Table 7-9 Trial Reliability Work Sheet for Tally and Duration Data

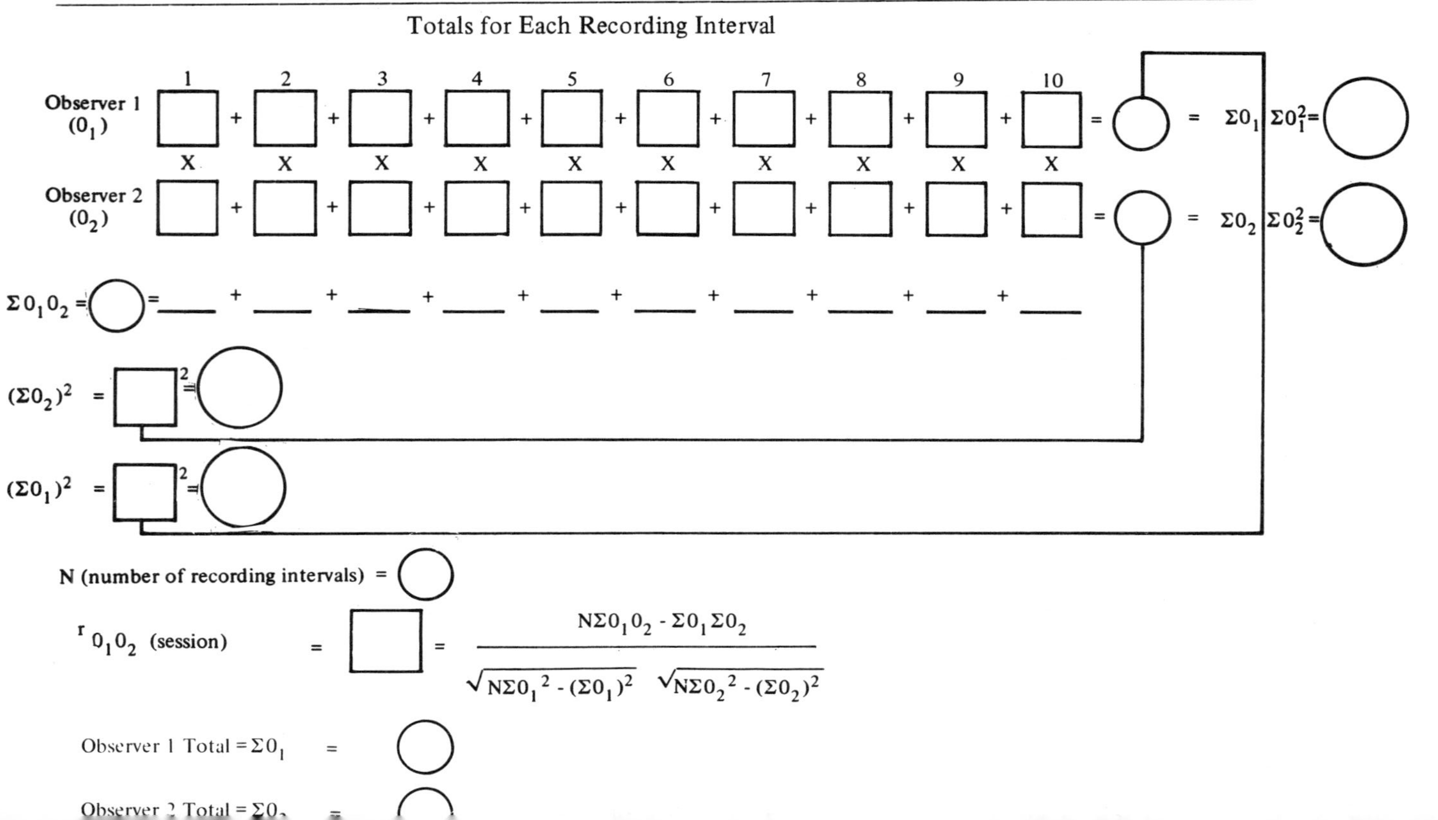

Interpreting and evaluating measures of trial interobserver reliability. It should be noted that the measure of reliability you have calculated is based on the scores obtained by dividing the data for a single session into a series of discrete intervals or trials. Thus, the measure of reliability indexes the consistency of the observers' ratings of the target behavior for these trials or intervals within a session. You will have occasion to repeat this procedure on other single sessions at least once each week or two during your project to check for "instrument decay" (Campbell and Stanley, 1963). These checks help insure that your scoring criteria remain consistent throughout the treatment program.

No entirely agreed upon set of rules for deciding on an acceptable level of reliability has yet been formulated. As a general principle, the reliability necessary for your study is dependent upon the degree of change in the target behavior you want to be able to demonstrate. To detect small changes produced by your treatment manipulation, reliability must be high. Gross changes, on the other hand, can be detected with even relatively unreliable measures.

You might want to use the rules of thumb we have developed for judging the adequacy of your data's reliability. For interval data, percentage agreement should be greater than 80% or r_{ϕ} should be greater than .6. For either the tally or duration method, $r_{0_1 0_2}$ should be greater than .6.

If the values you obtain fall below the recommended minimum, your first step is to do some trouble-shooting. Are your calculations correct? Are your definitions clear? (Perhaps you need to add more examples of positive and negative instances of the target behavior.) Were your timers synchronized? Was the child blocked from one of the observers' view for part of the time? Review the observation procedures recommended in Chapter 2. Whatever the problem is, try to remedy it, and collect another set of practice reliability data. If you still have problems with the second set of data, check with your instructor before you begin to collect formal baseline data.

Probe Questions for Part 2, Chapter 7

1. How will your choice of either the frequency, duration, or interval method of collecting data determine the number of data cells you have to work with?

2. What kinds of agreements and disagreements do the four cells in a two-by-two table include?

3. What methods are available for determining the reliability of occurrence-nonoccurrence data?

4. Why is it necessary to adjust data resulting from sessions of atypical length?

5. What action should be taken if your reliability estimates fall below acceptable standards?

6. Describe the advantages and limitations of percentage agreement, effective percentage agreement, and phi as measures of reliability for interval data.

Behavioral Objectives for Part 3, Chapter 7

After studying Part 3 of this chapter, you should be able to:

1. State the primary problems with the use of human observers.

2. Assess and evaluate observer drift.

3. Detect consensual observer drift.

Part 3. Observer Effects

OVERVIEW OF OBSERVER EFFECTS

Observer effects refer to changes in the data produced by the observers rather than by the treatment manipulation or independent variable. Johnson and Bolstad (1973), Rosenthal and Rosnow (1969), and Weick (1968) have catalogued and discussed the potential dangers of an apparently staggering number of these observer effects. The most widely recognized of these effects are discussed below.

Reactive Effects on the Child of Being Observed

The mere presence of an observer can produce changes in the child's behavior (see Chapter 2). Fortunately, these disruptive effects are probably most likely to occur during initial periods of observation and tend to dissipate with time as the child acclimates to the observer's presence. If these effects are present in your study, they would most likely affect the early baseline data. Therefore, you should compare your early baseline data with the data obtained at the end of baseline to see if such effects might be present. If the early and late baseline rates differ considerably, the observer's presence may have affected the child's behavior more at the inception of the study. Therefore, the later data points may be more representative of the child's baseline rate than are those obtained earlier during this phase.

Observer Bias

Observer bias is a wastebasket categorization that refers to a variety of factors that produce systematic observer inaccuracies. Included in this category are observer *expectancy effects,* or the unintentional selective misperception or miscoding of the target behavior because of the observer's hunches, guesses, or expectations about how the child should behave. Also included are consistent errors produced by other misapplications of the behavioral definitions, the coding system, the data sheets, or any other aspect of the data collection method.

While not all instances of observer bias can be ferreted out of your data, consistent *differences* between the degree of bias displayed by your two observers often can be detected. To do so, compare the two observers' totals for the target behavior after *each* reliability probe. If your totals disagree, work at trying to find out why. If you can't find the problem and you continue to disagree systematically on the totals (e.g., one observer regularly rates 10-15 percent more occurrences of the target behavior), it will be necessary to assign one observer the status of primary data gatherer; he will take data during each session while the remaining observer would be used only for reliability probes.

Also check at the conclusion of your study to see whether the session totals for the two observers in Table 7-9 are approximately the same across all of the joint observation sessions. If they differ by no more than a few points, no action need be taken. For larger discrepancies, the action required depends upon which of the following circumstances were in effect in your study.

1. If one observer has rated all sessions, his data should be used in the primary data analysis.

2. If two observers are used and neither one rates all of the sessions, check with your instructor. Changes in the child's behavior across conditions may be confounded with differences between observers across conditions.

3. If two observers rated all sessions, analyze the average of the two observers' data. Using two observers and pooling their ratings not only produces more reliable data but also avoids another observer effect, which we consider next.

Reactivity of the Observer to a Second Observer's Presence

Recent experiments by O'Leary and Kent (1973) and Reid (1970) have shown that the occasional presence of a reliability checker can have reactive effect. That is, an observer's data change systematically with the presence or absence of another person serving as a reliability checker. While there are other experiments that question the generality of this phenomenon (e.g., Whelan, 1974), it may be worthwhile to use two observers throughout the project if you are able conveniently to do so.

Observer Drift

The problem of detecting observer drift (that is, gradual changes in the criteria for a scorable response) may not be entirely solved by the ordinary reliability methods previously described. This is particularly true with the detection of gradual criteria changes by both observers – sometimes called consensual observer drift (Johnson and Bolstad, 1973). Gradual changes in both observers' criteria are particularly likely with a response such as "speech intelligibility." As the observers become more acquainted with the child's speech, the rated intelligibility increases – although the objective quality of the child's speech has not improved. A method that we have used to help detect this kind of observer "deterioration" is to record three or more tapes of the child's verbal behavior early in the study and have a third, trained observer rate these tapes. Then one tape is rated by the two usual observers at the beginning phases of the study, a second in the middle portion of the study, and third at the end of the study. If the latter tapes are rated higher by the two regular observers in comparison with the ratings made by the third observer, there are grounds for concern about downward drifting of criteria. For additional information on this method, see Gelfand, Hartmann, Lamb, Smith, Mahan, and Paul (1974) and Patterson and Harris (1968).

While it is better to detect than not to detect observer drift, bias, etc., it is better still to avoid these unwanted observer effects entirely. This is best accomplished by thorough and continuous training of the observers, maintenance of high observer morale, and attention to basic factors of human engineering.

CONCLUSIONS

The reliability procedures recommended in this chapter are fairly complex. To help you from getting lost in this complexity, we have summarized these procedures in a step-wise manner in Table 7-10. If you are collecting data on more than one target behavior, these procedures should be followed for each behavior.

Table 7-10 Step-by-Step Summary of Reliability Procedures

1. Both observers collect data during an observation session prior to formal baseline data collection. Check trial reliability and observer bias for each target behavior.
   (a) If summary data are unacceptable, troubleshoot problems and repeat Step 1.
   (b) If summary data are adequate, begin formal baseline data collection.
2. If necessary, construct material to assess observer drift.
3. Include trial reliability probes once each week or two, and at least once during each phase of the study. Check trial reliability and observer bias; resolve disagreements immediately following each reliability probe.
4. Summarize trial reliability data in Table 7-6.
5. Check for observer bias and drift over the entire course of the study.

To learn more about the intricacies of reliability theory, consult one of the standard references on the topic such as Guilford (1965, Chapter 17) or Nunnally (1967, Chapters 6 and 7). If you are specifically interested in the problems of reliability in behavior modification, check the recent papers by Hartmann, (1974, c), Herbert (1973), and Johnson and Bolstad (1973). Reliability methods based on the analysis of variance, and related to the correlation approach described in this chapter, are described in Winer (1971, Section 4.5), in Cronbach, Gleser, Nanda, and Rajaratnam (1972), in Medley and Mitzel (1963), and in Wiggins (1973).

Probe Questions for Part 3, Chapter 7

1. Distinguish between the two types of reactive effects (on the child and on the observer in the presence of a second observer) discussed in this section.

2. What is observer bias? How might observer bias pose a problem in interpreting your results?

3. How might failure to detect consensual observer drift affect the evaluation of the effectiveness of a treatment program?

Behavioral Objectives for Part 1, Chapter 8

After studying Part 1 of this chapter, you should be able to:

1. State the advantages of keeping up-to-date graphs of the target behavior's rate.

2. Determine the length of the baseline phase of your study.

3. State the advantages and disadvantages of grouping your data.

CHAPTER 8

Formal Data Collection

Part 1. Collecting Baseline Data

INTRODUCTION

You should have now completed all the steps leading up to formal data collection. Your definitions have been refined, a smoothly functioning data collection method has been developed and tested, and minor reliability problems have been resolved. Now use your observation and recording techniques to collect a record of the child's rate of responding. As your study passes from one phase to the next, continue to collect data on the target behavior. Before you begin collecting data each day, review the Data Collection Checklist presented in Table 8-1; it may keep you from making some easily avoidable errors. When you have completed your daily observations, summarize them by tabulating occurrences of the target behavior in the Data Summary Table (see Table 7-6) as well as on a working graph. (Specific details on the construction of graphs are found in Chapter 10.) We found that a daily graphic record of the rate of the target behavior has a number of advantages. First, a well-constructed graph will allow you to determine at a glance whether changes should be made in your treatment program and whether it is time to move to the next stage of your experimental design. Second, a simple, easily interpreted graph can be used to provide feedback and reinforcement to the child's caretakers, and perhaps to the child himself (see Chapter 3, Part 1).

Table 8-1 Data Collection Checklist

1.______ Have you rechecked the behavioral definitions, including definitions of positive and negative instances?

2.______ Is the equipment needed for taking data (pencils, stopwatches, data sheets) available? (For both observers, if it's a reliability probe.)

3.______ Be sure your data sheets are dated and otherwise labeled. If this is a reliability probe, also staple the two data sheets together after you have completed your observations.

4.______ If your reliability wasn't too good on the last probe, discuss your errors, and include another reliability probe.

5.______ Do you have enough data during this condition? Remember, if you plan to group your data, for example, plot them weekly rather than daily, the number of required daily observations is greater than if you do not group your data.

6.______ Have you included a reliability check within the past five-to-six days? If not, include another reliability probe. If you have more than one target behavior, be certain to check the reliability of each one.

COLLECTING BASELINE DATA

Formal data collection will begin during the baseline condition. In this condition you will obtain a record of the child's naturally occurring, baseline rate of responding. This rate will be compared with rates of the behavior during treatment and other subsequent conditions so that the degree of change can be determined and the variables responsible for this change can be identified.

Length of Baseline Phase

Continue collecting baseline data until you either obtain a stable rate of responding or until you are confident that the behavior is not consistently changing in the desired direction even without your intervention. The length of baseline will then depend upon the rate, variability, and direction of change in the target behavior, and upon some reality factors such as length of the school term in which you are to complete your project.

In addition, the length of baseline, as well as the succeeding phases of your study, will depend upon whether or not you intend to use formal statistical analysis. Jones, Vaught, and Reid (1973) suggest a minimum of ten data points within each condition if time series analyses are to be performed on the data. Hartmann (1974, d) recommends a minimum of 12 stable data points within each condition if analysis of variance procedures are to be performed on the data.

Baseline rate varies from day to day, but varies around a discernible average rate. Sidman (1960) recommends that a stable baseline should not vary more than five percent. That is a reasonable value for a rat in a Skinner box, but unreasonable for a child in a complex and varying social environment. Rather than striving for some high level of stability achievable in only the most controlled of laboratory situations, we recommend that you: (1) examine the factors that produce variability – this may help you to generate a successful treatment strategy; and (2) evaluate your baseline from the standpoint of its regularity, rather than just its stability – that is, a child may show a high rate of refusal to eat each weekend, but a low rate during the week. A resulting graph of this response (refusing food) might show great regularity from week to week but little apparent stability from day to day. Recognition of this pattern requires a more extended observation period than is necessary when the rate is zero or is quite stable. Cyclic data of this type are shown in Fig. 8-1: If baseline data collection would have been terminated

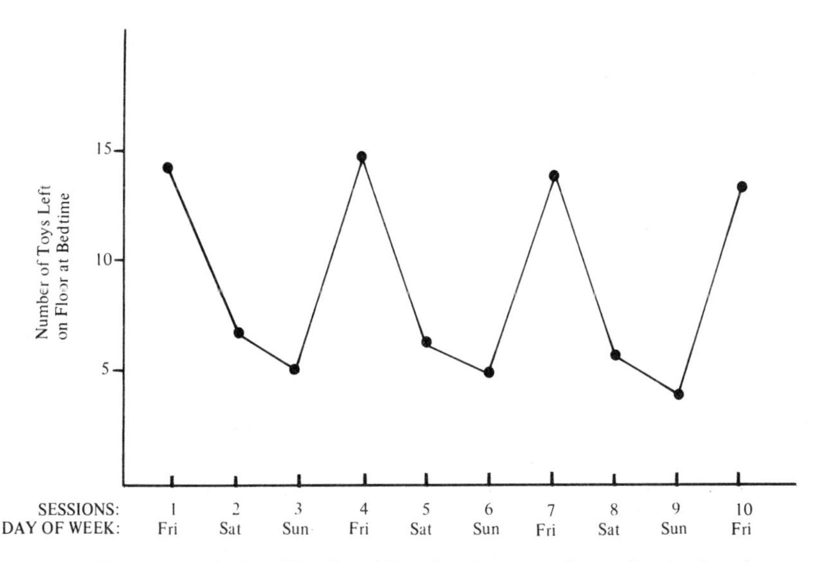

Fig. 8-1. Example of a baseline in which the data vary from day to day, but vary around a discernible average and in a stable weekly pattern.

at Day 4, no notion of the regularity of the data would have been obtained. Data with recurring cycles such as these are more often seen in weekly cycles – i.e., the rates of the behavior are discriminated on the day of the week, so that room-cleaning might be very low in rate on weekdays and much higher on weekends. In order to clarify these weekly cycles, be sure to label the horizontal axis of your baseline graph with the day of the week on which each data point was obtained.

If your data are variable, use the following rule of thumb to decide how many baseline sessions to include: three plus one additional day for each ten percent of variability – that is: Number of days of baseline = 3+10 [(Highest Rate – Lowest Rate)/Highest Rate]. For example, if the number of homework problems solved varies from six to 20 during the first three days of baseline, continue to take baseline data for seven additional days – 10[(20-6)/20]=7. This rule of thumb for determining the length of baseline is for use when one's schedule is under the control of data – an admirable criterion, but one that we only infrequently can afford. It will probably be necessary for you to keep uppermost in mind the constraints imposed by academic scheduling. If too much time is spent collecting baseline data, it might then be necessary to skimp on either the treatment or other phases of your study, which in the long run might have greater importance.

Once the baseline data appear orderly, consult with your instructor before proceeding with the treatment program; your assessment of stability may be premature. The baseline data shown in Panel A of Fig. 8-2 could be considered sufficiently stable to begin treatment; the mean number of room-cleaning items completed is 17, with scores ranging from 15-18.

The baseline data presented in Panel B of Fig. 8-2 are not sufficiently stable to begin modifying the behavior. The rate of food requests including "please" varies from 15% to 55% with a mean of 27%; an additional six or seven days of baseline data should be obtained. At the end of that time, the data may become more stable, or at least the factors that produce extensive variability may become apparent.

A technique sometimes used to reduce the apparent variability in a set of data is to group the data across larger time intervals. Instead of grouping the data across the recording intervals during a single session and plotting daily session totals, one could average and graph the data for a number of days, perhaps even a week. This procedure has much to recommend it as a method of producing apparent clarity where before there was only chaos. On the other hand, grouping data may disguise controlling factors that could be discerned with ungrouped data, and also usually requires additional data. For example, if data were grouped or collapsed over five day averages, a minimum of ten days of data would be required for two data points.

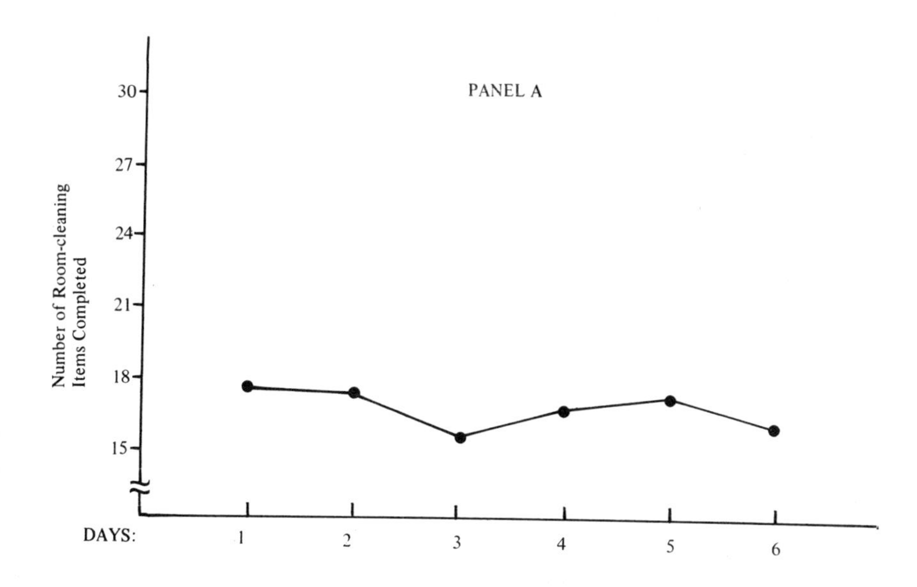

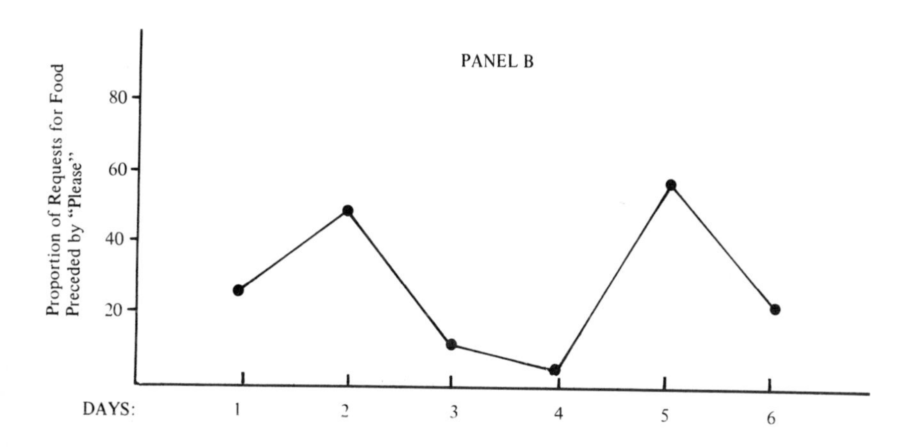

Fig. 8-2. Examples of variable (Panel B) and stable (Panel A) baselines.

As an aid to understanding your data, you may find it useful to construct one graph of daily session totals and a second graph of totals averaged over several days or some other convenient period of time.

Baseline rate is shifting progressively from day to day. It is acceptable to initiate a program when the direction of progressive shift is opposite to the change direction desired. Panel A of Fig. 8-3 shows a baseline appropriate for beginning a deceleration program. Although the rate of thumb-sucking is on the increase, continual increases will work against rather than in the direction of your program. As a result of beginning on the upswing, you will underestimate the potency of your program. (Part of the scientific tradition is that if you must err, do so conservatively. This is another example of scientists' reinforcement schedules being thinned by institutionalized practices.) You would not want to begin an acceleration program with the target behavior on the

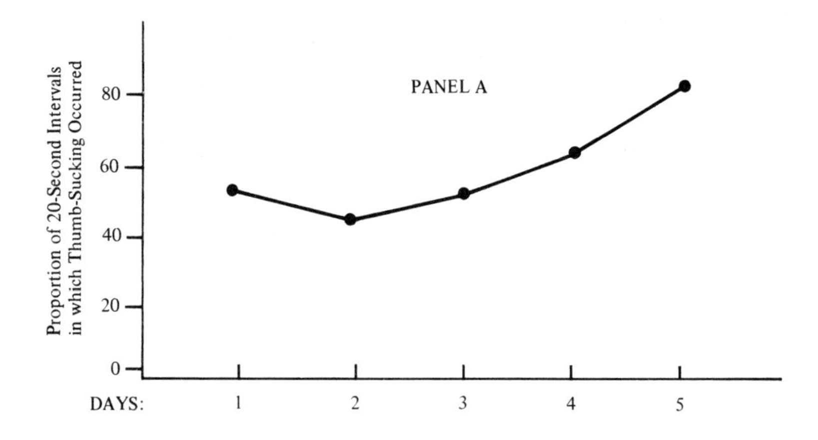

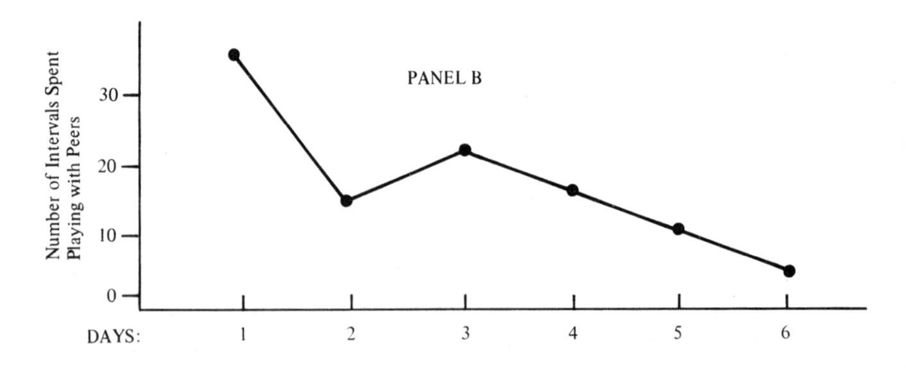

Fig. 8-3. Example of accelerating (Panel A) and decelerating (Panel B) baselines.

increase. If your baseline looked like the one for time spent interacting with peers (presented in Panel B of Fig. 8-3), it would be appropriate for you to begin an acceleration program but not a deceleration program.

When the shift is in the desired direction, but very gradual, you may begin your modification program. The baseline rate of minutes crying before afternoon nap (shown in Fig. 8-4) provides just such an example. Although the rate is decreasing, it is doing so at a very slow rate; if your program is successful, you should substantially decrease the rate. If you are able to do so, check into the factors that are responsible for the decreasing baseline rate; they may suggest a method of controlling the behavior.

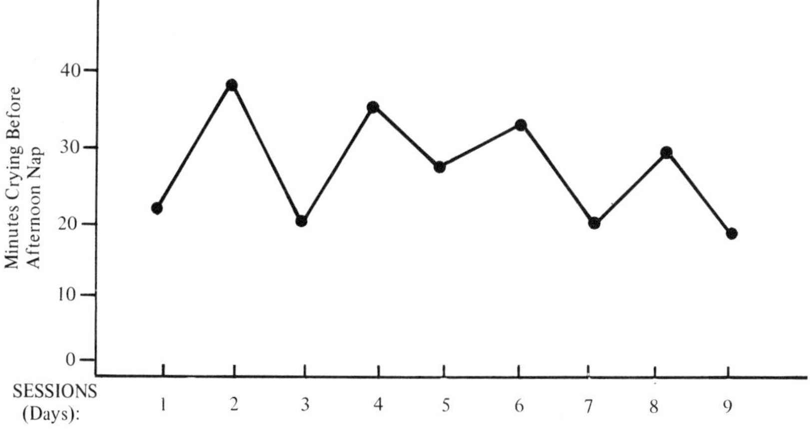

Fig. 8-4. Example of a gradually decreasing baseline.

When the shift is dramatic and in the desired direction, it may be unnecessary for you to add a separate therapeutic manipulation. Someone or something else is effectively modifying the behavior. You had best select another behavior for modification. Perhaps your observation is a reactive measure – e.g., the teacher knows what behavior you are observing and she begins to respond differently to that behavior with a resulting impact on its rate, or the child realizes that his table manners are annoying others so he initiates some self-control procedures. Unanticipated changes of this sort are a boon to the child, but perhaps temporarily disappointing to you because of the time you have invested in the project. Perhaps all is not lost, however, if you select another target behavior for modification with the same child. Like adults, few children are perfect.

Zero rate of a desirable target behavior. This circumstance makes a formal and extended period of baseline observation virtually unnecessary. The baseline rate is, has been, and probably will remain at zero – e.g., the child has never made his bed. If so, you can commence with your behavior modification program. (See Part 2 of Chapter 4.)

Multiple baseline designs. With multiple baseline designs, the principles described above should be applied to the baseline of each of the two or more target behaviors. If one of the behaviors is markedly unstable, begin treatment with one of the more stable behaviors. Because there is some slight risk in beginning treatment before all of the target responses have stabilized, check with your instructor.

Problems with baseline data. A number of problems can occur with your data even at this early stage of your study. Following are some of the most likely problems and their solutions:

1. The baseline is rising prior to beginning an acceleration program (or falling prior to beginning a deceleration program).
   Solution: Hold tight! Wait until the baseline rate stabilizes. If it continues to increase, you may have achieved a "baseline cure," and you can move on to the treatment of some other problem behavior.
2. Poor observer reliability. The effect of poor observer reliability is often to obscure any treatment effects. The resulting data are likely to be quite noisy with no obvious differences between conditions. (See the data in Fig. 8-5 for an example of how the data might look from an entire study conducted with poor reliability.)

   Solution: The solution is obvious – improve your reliability. If you've tried that without success, you may also want to use as data the average of the two observers' ratings. That means that *each* session will have to be rated by both observers, which is not always possible. (As noted in Chapter 7, the average of two ratings will be more reliable than the ratings of a single rater.) Sometimes choppy data occur even when the raters agree – the child is simply variable from day to day. Occasionally, extending the conditions may give you clues concerning the cause of variability, and that may suggest appropriate remedial action. At other times, the best strategy is simply to average the data over two, three, or even more sessions. Possibly, by doing so, the "random" variations in the behavior will wash out.

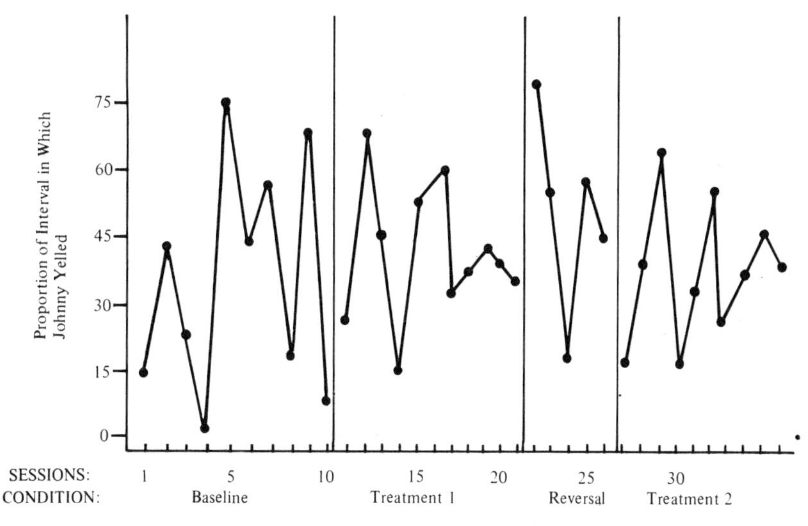

Fig. 8-5. Graph showing very "noisy," uninterpretable data, perhaps arising from low observer reliability.

Generalization Probes

If your study is one in which generalization probes would be useful (e.g., training occurs for a very limited portion of the day, and the behavior is relevant to a much wider variety of contexts), you should begin gathering baseline data in those situations in which you wish to test for generalization (see Part 3 of Chapter 3 and Part 1 of Chapter 9). Again, the rules regarding stability, etc. are applicable to evaluating the baseline data collected during generalization probes. However, if generalization is only a minor focus of your study, it may be acceptable to include weekly rather than daily generalization probes and bend the rules concerning stability. Check with your instructor.

Conclusions

When you have collected sufficient baseline data – that is, the data are regular, reliable, and not changing in the treatment-aimed direction – begin the treatment manipulation. If you are doubtful about the appropriateness of beginning treatment, check with your instructor.

Note: Each day you collect data be certain to review Table 8-1, the Data Collection Checklist, and then summarize your data in a Data Summary Table and on a working graph.

Probe Questions for Part 1, Chapter 8

1. What are the advantages of maintaining a graph of your data throughout the study?

2. Before moving from the baseline to the treatment phase of your study, what criteria regarding stability, trends, and grouping of data should be fulfilled?

3. The baseline rate of food-throwing for a two-year-old boy over the course of six consecutive days is as follows: 23%, 16%, 18%, 13%, and 10%. Comment on the advisability of beginning a deceleration program at this point.

4. Distinguish between a regular and a stable baseline.

Behavioral Objectives for Part 2, Chapter 8

After studying this section, you should be able to:

1. State the criteria for terminating the treatment phase of your study.

2. Determine the length of each subsequent phase of your study.

3. Solve problems that commonly occur during the treatment and subsequent phases of your study.

Part 2. Collecting Data During Treatment and Follow-Up

COLLECTING DATA DURING TREATMENT

Continue to collect data throughout the treatment phase of your study. If you have included generalization probes, also collect generalization data during treatment. If you are conducting a multiple baseline study, continue to collect baseline data on the nonmanipulated behaviors as well as the behavior that is presently undergoing modification.

Length of Treatment Manipulation

There are two formal criteria that should be considered in determining the length of your treatment manipulation: the social relevance criterion and the scientific criterion. In addition, the matter of expediency and your (or the child's) academic requirements may help determine your project's duration.

The social relevance criterion. Has the rate of the target behavior been changed sufficiently so that the child is no longer considered atypical when compared to his same-aged peers? Are the child and his caretakers satisfied with the change produced? For example, if the target behavior was thumb-sucking, the rate should be lowered sufficiently so that the behavior is no longer of concern to the child's caretakers. If, instead, you worked with an acceleration problem, such as taking-out-the-garbage, the rate should be sufficiently high that the child's caretakers would agree that the performance is now thoroughly acceptable. Although the social relevance criterion is not the only one for determining length of treatment, it is certainly an important consideration; unless it is met, treatment should not be terminated without good reason.

The scientific criterion. Has the behavior been changed sufficiently so that any reasonable person examining a graph of the rate of the behavior would agree that the behavior has been changed? This criterion implies that, in comparison to the baseline rate, the treatment rate has *stabilized* at a new and discernibly different rate. Methods of determining stability are discussed in Part 1 of this chapter; formal rules for determining change are presented in Chapter 10.

Occasionally, the social relevance criterion is apparently met (i.e., the child's caretakers agree that the problem no longer exists), but the data fail to substantiate their claim. When this occurs, continue treatment until the reports by caretakers and your data are congruent. If the data indicate changes in the target behavior, but the caretakers report no change, check with your instructor as to how to proceed.

Occasionally, the two criteria described above are not completely satisfied, but time for completing your study is running short; extension of the treatment phase might then sacrifice the remaining portions of your study. If you face this dilemma, consult with your instructor. If you are using a reversal design, he may suggest that you abbreviate Treatment 1 and the reversal phase, and lengthen Treatment 2. With the initially treated behavior in a multiple baseline design, the two criteria may be relaxed slightly, as you can continue modification of the first target response while you are applying the treatment to the remaining target responses.

Problems

Again there are a number of problems that might occur during the treatment portion of your study. Some of these problems and their solutions are given below.

1. The rate during treatment continues to change.
   Solution: If the rate has clearly changed in the desired direction, there is no basis for concern. Simply institute the next condition. If the rate falls after an initial rise, it might be that the behavior was being controlled by some extratherapeutic factor. Or perhaps the child is satiating on whatever reinforcer is being used. Continue the treatment sessions a bit longer to see what will happen, and read Chapter 5 carefully for other suggestions.
2. Nonindependent behaviors or situations in a multiple baseline design. If you look carefully at the multiple baseline data in Fig. 8-6, you'll notice something peculiar. When treatment was instituted for setting the lunch table, that behavior improved – but so did setting the breakfast and the dinner table. We might optimistically say that the treatment generalized to the other conditions. Obviously then, the three stimulus situations were not independent. A skeptic might say that there is no demonstration that the treatment changed the behavior; and he is, of course, correct. Some concomitant event not included in the treatment program might just as well have been responsible for the behavior change. Without further information, the two alternative interpretations seem equally compelling. Although the target behavior is undoubtedly changed, we can't specify what is responsible for the change.
   Solution: If you find an upward drift in all behaviors following institution of treatment for the first behavior in a multiple baseline design, you might superimpose a reversal phase. If this does not seem to be a reasonable tactic, check with your instructor.

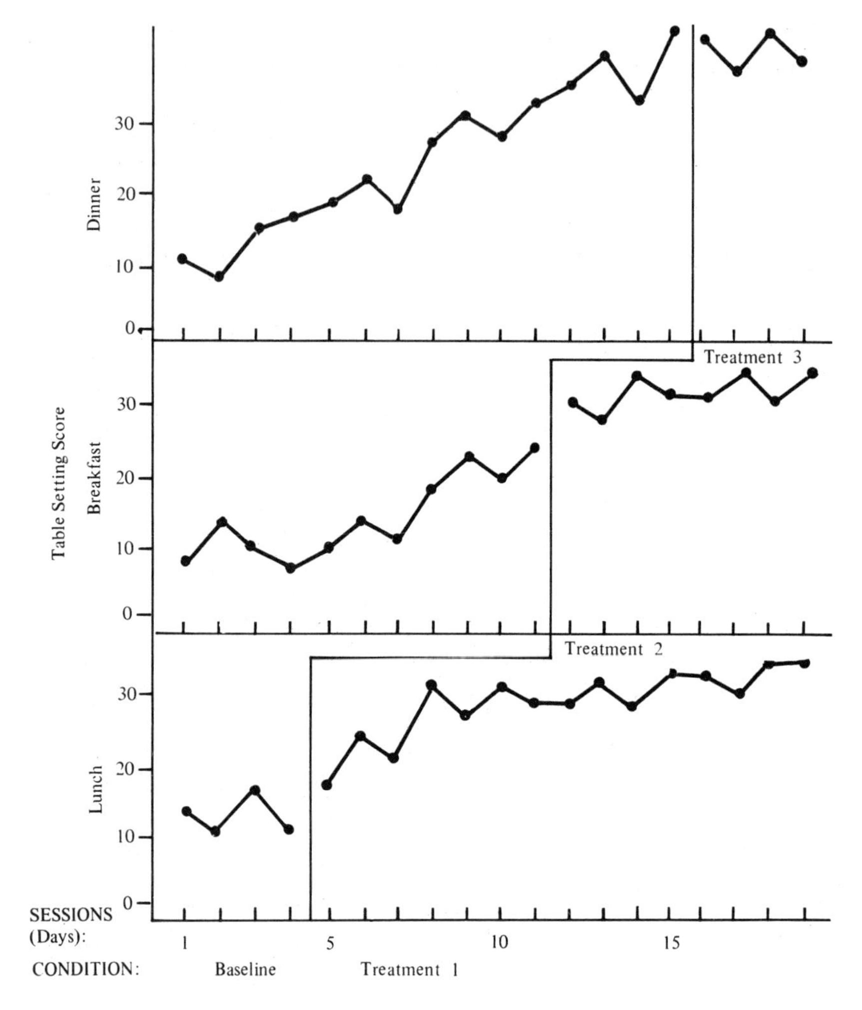

Fig. 8-6. Data showing the failure of a multiple baseline design to demonstrate experimental control because of the nonindependence of the three behaviors.

3. On occasion, students – and professionals as well – simply cannot modify a behavior. Sometimes target behaviors are strongly under the control of variables that themselves are not readily amenable to change. At other times, a correct treatment technique is not

employed until too late in the project. At still other times, no effective treatment is available. In all of these situations, the data look like a greatly extended baseline – no changes observed, no control over the behavior. In such situations one can often say nothing with certainty except that the behavior was untreatable with the techniques used.

Solution: There is really no very acceptable solution for such a problem. If time allows, you may, of course, attempt other treatment techniques. If that is impossible, sometimes careful scrutiny of the data in comparison with a retrospective diary of concomitant changes in the child's life may produce some useful hypothesis that can be tested at a later time. Tukey (1970) suggests various methods that can be applied in exploratory data analysis.

Even failure can have its advantages, because inadequacy of our present set of treatment techniques may spur the search for new and more effective ones.

Conclusion

If careful inspection of your data and the report of the child's caretakers indicate that the target behavior has been successfully modified, go on to the next stage in your study. If you are uncertain about when to institute the next phase of your study, check with your instructor.

COLLECTING DATA IN THE REMAINING PHASES OF YOUR STUDY

The general rules for determining the length of each succeeding phase of your study are the same as those already described, with one exception: the length of the reversal phase in an ABAB design is often abbreviated because of the inconvenience associated with returning a behavior to an undesirable rate. You should, however, have a sufficient number of data points during the reversal phase so that any reasonable person would agree that a real change in the rate has occurred, though the rate may not have stabilized. Again, the rules for determining change are described in Chapters 7 and 10.

Note: Be sure to continue your generalization probes. Also continue to review the Data Collection Checklist and to use the Data Summary Sheet and a daily graph.

Problems

We again describe for you a number of problems that may first become apparent during the later steps of your study, and offer some suggestions for solving these problems.

1. Treatment-by-observer confounding. The data presented in Fig. 8-7 illustrate a major flaw in an N=1 study. The mother was the principal data gatherer during baseline and reversal, while the daughter took data during the two treatment phases. When the reliability data were examined carefully, it was found that the mother had consistently higher rates, higher by 30 percent on the average. What seems to be a clear-cut treatment effect might instead be nothing but differences in the observers.
Solution: Obviously the best solution for treatment-by-observer confounding is to avoid it by carefully noting any tendency of the observers to differ in their totals early in the study and either resolve the problem or use one observer as the primary data gatherer. If you have been inattentive to signs of observer bias early in the study and find yourself with data like those shown in Fig. 8-7, you may still be able to save your project. If there is a fairly consistent trend for one observer to see more of the target

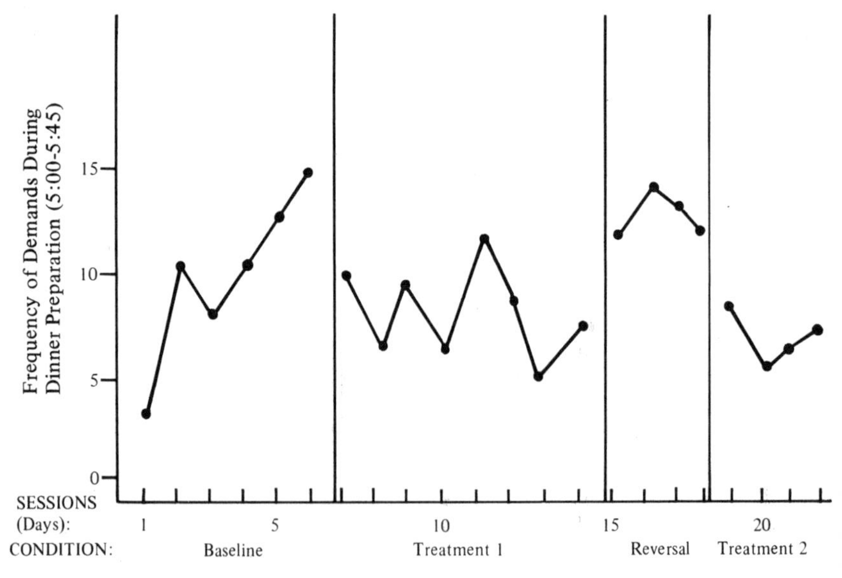

Fig. 8-7. Data during baseline and reversal conditions, obtained by mother, and those during treatments 1 and 2 obtained by daughter. Differences bet conditions are thus confounded with differences between observers.

behavior than the other, you might subtract that constant quantity from the higher observer's data when you prepare your final graph. Before taking such drastic action, check with your instructor. If he approves of it, be sure to note any modifications of the data of this sort on your graph, and provide your justification for manipulating the data in the text of your final report.

2. Inability to recapture baseline. An examination of the reversal phase of the data presented in Fig. 8-8 clearly indicates that the baseline rate could not be recaptured, and hence there was no

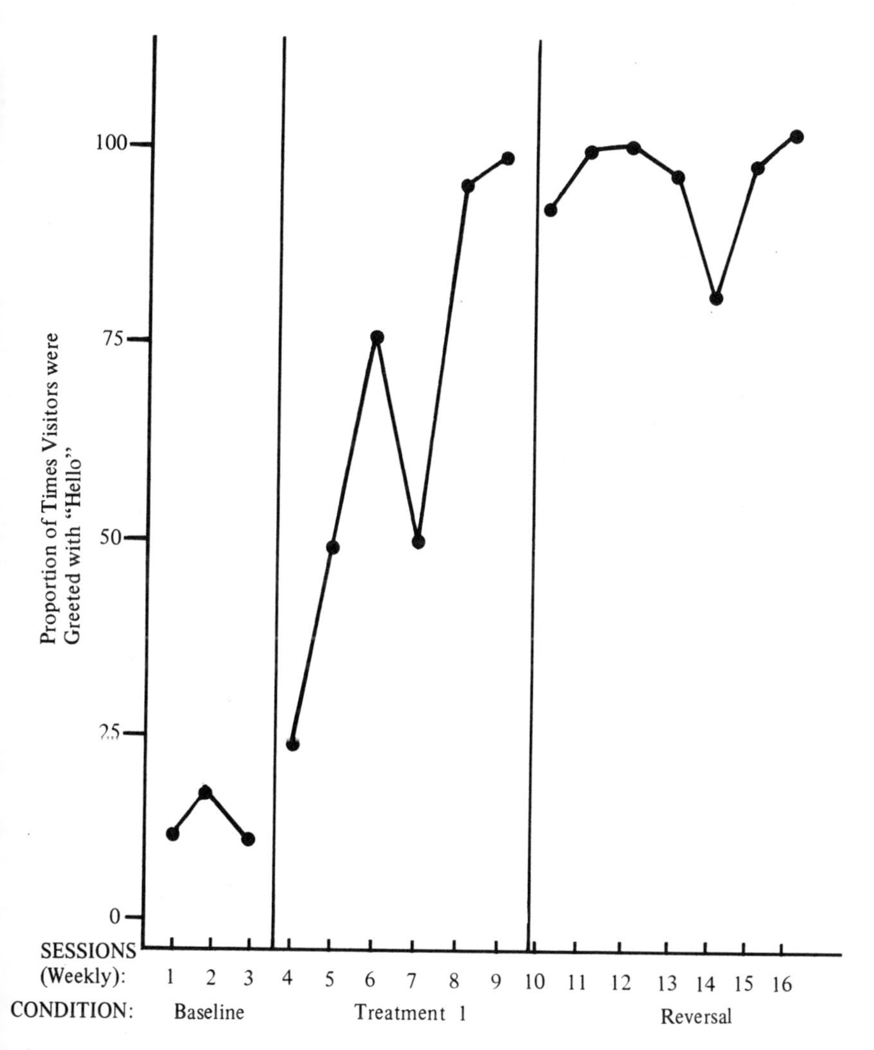

Fig. 8-8. Graph showing the failure of a reversal condition to recapture baseline rates.

opportunity to demonstrate control by repeatedly turning the behavior on and off by putting in and taking out the treatment variable. We might speculate that perhaps the child was obtaining generous social reinforcement for his new social skills outside of the home, and that this reinforcement was sufficient to maintain the behavior at home even when it was put on extinction.
A solution: If time enough remains, add a DRO condition (see Part 2 of Chapter 4 and Part 1 of Chapter 6), then remove the DRO when the behavior has decreased. If the rate of behavior remains low (stabilizes), reinstitute the treatment. If the behavior remains unaffected by either the DRO or other decelerating procedures, you may be able to add certain components of a multiple baseline strategy; discuss this problem with your instructor.

COLLECTING DATA DURING FOLLOW-UP

If time is still available, wait two to six weeks after the completion of the last stage of your project, and check the durability of the therapeutic changes by collecting follow-up data. Follow-up data are usually taken under natural maintaining conditions; the data are collected in the same situations as they were during the treatment proper, and under whatever maintaining conditions presently exist (see Part 3 of Chapter 3).

After you have completed data collection and tabulation during all phases of your study (possibly including generalization probes and follow-up), you will be ready to analyze your data. The procedures to be followed are described in Chapter 10.

Probe Questions for Part 2, Chapter 8

1. Why might it be unwise to terminate the treatment phase of a study before the social relevance and scientific criteria are met?

2. What are some of the data collection problems that might occur during the treatment phase of a study? How might these problems be solved?

3. Define treatment-by-observer confounding. Describe the potential remedies for this problem.

4. If the baseline rate of the target behavior cannot be recaptured in an ABAB design by reinstituting the conditions present during baseline, what procedures might be employed to demonstrate experimental control?

Behavioral Objectives for Part 1, Chapter 9

Study of Part 1 of this chapter should equip you to:

1. Say why one should avoid large-magnitude, abrupt reductions in the frequency of reinforcement given a child for his desirable behavior.

2. Devise a plan to reduce the child's reliance on frequent and immediate reinforcement, but still maintain his newly acquired, prosocial performance.

3. Avoid inadvertently teaching the child to behave well only in your presence or only in the treatment setting.

4. Train the child's caretakers to conduct the treatment program, if appropriate.

5. Say why it is important to gain some control over the behavior of the child's playmates, and describe methods for doing so.

CHAPTER 9

Phasing Out and Concluding the Program

Part 1. Increasing Treatment Effect Generalization and Durability by Varying Reinforcers, Schedules, Treatment Agents, and Settings

This chapter describes a series of manipulations that might help promote the durability and generality of treatment effects. The modification of a target-problem behavior is no mean feat in itself, requiring ingenuity, persistence, and good judgment. Therefore, it is almost too much to expect a student therapist also to insure that the child's behavioral improvements are both general and enduring. We offer suggestions for the accomplishment of this latter task with the understanding that many students will not have the opportunity to extend and continue their treatment programs in this manner. Nevertheless, they may wish to know what could be done, and they may be able to undertake such procedures in the future.

Preventing the client's behavior from reverting to pretreatment patterns soon after the cessation of treatment is one of the most formidable tasks associated with behavior modification programs. If such a reversion were to occur, the client would have benefitted only briefly from the program; and he and his family might become unduly pessimistic about the possibility of his ever improving. In other words, in some instances a speedy relapse might worsen an initially unfortunate situation.

Another type of problem occurs when treatment effects are highly specific and situation-bound. It is entirely possible that the treatment you employ in the child's classroom durably improves his behavior in that environment but nowhere else. So he might behave like an angel in the treatment situation, but exhibit no improvement at other times and places. In this instance, again, the treatment would not have helped him very much.

This chapter describes a number of steps you can take to increase the durability and generality of the treatment effects. For example, multiple change agents and training settings might be introduced. Or you might thin the reinforcement schedules maintaining the child's desirable behavior so that the transition to naturally occurring schedules is less abrupt; you might also introduce reinforcing stimuli most likely to be found in his everyday life. Other possibilities include transferring the administration of the modification program to the child's caretakers, to his age-mates, and to the child himself, if possible. Each of these techniques will be described in some detail in this chapter. Most of these methods require considerable planning and implementation time, so you should make your decision regarding their use well in advance of your anticipated program termination date.

ALTER REINFORCEMENT SCHEDULES

An abrupt transition from a rich reinforcement procedure in the modification program to a posttreatment situation in which no provision is made for the administration of reinforcers is often tantamount to placing the desired target behavior on an extinction schedule. In such circumstances, a return to the original, unsatisfactory behavior patterns is highly predictable (Davison and Taffel, 1972; O'Leary and Drabman, 1971; Patterson, McNeal, Hawkins, and Phelps, 1967; Walker, Mattson, and Buckley, 1971). Instead, reinforcement schedule transitions must be introduced gradually over a period of time in order to avoid the performance loss resulting from changing suddenly from a very rich reinforcement schedule to a very lean one (Ferster and Perrott, 1968; Ferster and Skinner, 1957). The wise therapist incorporates increasing intermittency of reinforcement into the treatment whenever circumstances permit. The process of thinning and discontinuing therapeutic reinforcement contingencies has also been discussed in Part 2 of Chapter 5. We reiterate this aspect of contingency management here because of its importance in the maintenance of improved behavior after the treatment intervention has been terminated.

Implementation

If you have been applying a fixed-interval or fixed-ratio schedule, introduce a less predictable variable schedule prior to termination. The variable schedule more nearly matches most naturally occurring schedules (Ferster and Perrott, 1968) and so blends well into the child's everyday routine. If you have applied a variable schedule since the inception of treatment, increase its intermittency until the natural environment's schedule is closely approximated. As we mentioned previously, it is advisable to thin the schedule gradually. Sometimes the process of thinning the reinforcement schedule produces a performance loss. This problem is relatively easily remedied, however. Should the target behavior decrease appreciably in rate following an increase in performance requirements to earn each reinforcer, you must revert to the immediately preceding schedule, restabilize this behavior, and then introduce a less dramatic schedule change. (Note that this procedure is similar to that employed whenever introduction of a new performance requirement disrupts the process of shaping.) Insofar as possible, avoid large magnitude and sudden reductions in the frequency of reinforcement of the desired behavior.

Murdock and Hartmann (in press) recommend the delivery of social reinforcers on a CRF schedule during language training programs and delivery of tangible reinforcers on a gradually thinned schedule beginning at CRF until the child reaches a criterion of 80 percent or more correct responding for two consecutive training sessions. Next, tangible reinforcers are administered for every second correct response (an FR2 schedule). If responding is maintained at the 80 percent level, the reinforcement is administered on the more intermittent, less predictable variable ratio schedule, such as a VR5. Eventually, social reinforcement could be made increasingly intermittent and tangible reinforcers could be completely eliminated.

OTHER ASPECTS OF CONTINGENCY MANAGEMENT

Two other transition operations that enhance durability of treatment effects have also been previously presented in Part 2 of Chapter 5. Consequently, we will only briefly restate them here. These procedures are the introduction of an increasing delay in the administration of back-up reinforcers and the introduction of varied, naturalistic reinforcers. Some delay between a target performance and receiving the back-up reinforcer such as monetary payment is characteristic of real life. Thus, if delay has been made a part of the treatment intervention, there is less disjunction, and hence less disruption in performance when the child returns to the naturalistic situation.

In addition, the child may infrequently encounter the types of reinforcers in his everyday life that are used in the treatment program. Therefore, the therapist should determine the nature of the reinforcers usually administered by the child's caretakers. Then these reinforcers should be utilized in the termination phase of the treatment program. These two procedures – delay of back-up reinforcers and introduction of naturalistic reinforcers – should help promote lasting changes in the child's behavior.

VARY CHANGE AGENTS AND THERAPY SETTINGS

Individuals can come to serve as S^D's for particular appropriate and inappropriate behaviors. Thus, the presence of peers might set the occasion for high-rate aggressive play, while adults signal the appropriateness of non-aggressive behavior (Martin, Gelfand, and Hartmann, 1971). Similarly, a particular classmate might occasion precise articulation, but another child might not (Johnston and Johnston, 1972). In treatment situations, there is the possibility of the therapist's becoming discriminative for his client's reinforcement for appropriate behavior. This problem seems to occur most acutely when aversive control procedures are employed (see Risley, 1968), but it is also associated with the application of positive behavior modification techniques. Since it is patently impossible for the therapist to remain with the child all of the time, he must take steps to insure that stimuli other than his presence come to act as S^D's for the child's desirable behaviors. Likewise, he must ward against a particular treatment location's becoming discriminative for the child's proper conduct.

The research literature on generalization and transfer of training offers bases for a number of possible remedies (Deese and Hulse, 1967, Chapter 10; Kimble, 1961, Chapter 11). The findings indicate that, in general, the greater the similarity between the training and the nontraining environments, the greater the transfer of training from one setting to the other. These considerations suggest the following procedures:

1. More than one change agent should be used in order to prevent the child from discriminating too closely on the trainer's presence (Goldstein, Heller, and Sechrest, 1966, Chapter 5). Since you are probably working with a partner as we have advised, you and your partner can easily meet this requirement by alternating as behavior managers. Employment of the child's family and friends as change agents further increases the probability of generality and maintenance of treatment effects, as will be discussed in following sections.

2. Training sessions should not be restricted to individual instruction with one therapist and one child. Instead, group size should be increased by small increments to approximate the social conditions the child will later encounter. Koegel and Rincover (1973) have discovered that skills mastered by autistic children in one-to-one instruction fail to generalize to group instruction settings. The children did not display the behaviors they had been

taught individually even when they were placed in groups as small as two children with one teacher. In contrast, a training procedure that employed a gradual increase in group size coupled with increasing intermittency of reinforcement enabled the children to continue their improved performance in a classroom of eight children with one teacher. Less deviant children may, however, require less generalization training than do autistic or very retarded youngsters.

3. Therapeutic training should be conducted in a number of different settings rather than in just one (Goldstein, Heller, and Sechrest, 1966, Chapter 5; Kazdin and Bootzin, 1972). Initially, it might be most advantageous to conduct each session in the same location at the same time of day. (The rationale for employing unvarying treatment settings and times is offered in Chapters 3, 8, and 10.) Toward the conclusion of treatment, however, considerations concerning the transfer and maintenance of the improved behavior would dictate some variation in training locale.

Some therapists have put this principle into practice. Goocher and Ebner (1968), for example, systematically introduced more complex, varied, and distracting settings while continuing to reinforce a child's appropriate classroom behaviors (e.g., attending to the teacher and to assigned work). The settings used began with the experimenter and child alone in a room and ended with the child in his classroom with the other children. The introduction of each new training setting temporarily disrupted the child's performance, but his appropriate academic behavior persisted after training was discontinued.

If time permits, then, we recommend that you use a number of different behavior managers and a variety of training settings. These practices will promote the transfer of treatment effects to natural environment settings and enhance their persistence following treatment termination. The following section by Murdock and Hartmann (in press) describes procedures designed to test for and to train generalization of speech skills.

> Language generalization requires that the child be able to respond correctly on all language tasks which he has mastered with the language instructor (1) in other physical settings, (2) for other people, (3) to different discriminative stimuli and (4) to similar language tasks. For example, assume the language instructor [therapist] is working with the child in an isolated therapy booth. The instructor points to a picture of the child's mother and asks, "Who is this?" The child responds correctly, "Mama." In order to have all four kinds of generalization, the child would also have to respond correctly (1) to the same picture and question when asked in other physical settings, e.g., classroom or home, (2) to the same picture and question when asked by someone other than the language instructor, (3) to the actual mother rather than a picture of his mother when asked the identical question or a variation of the

question, and (4) to be able to utilize his mastery of the "m ' phoneme to form other words, e.g., mom, me, and my.

A. *Generalization Probing.* Probing, i.e., testing for generalization, should be done for each task as soon as the child succeeds 80% or better on a VR5 schedule for two consecutive sessions with the language instructor. In order to determine whether the child's language behaviors are generalizing, the language instructor should set up probes to test for each kind of generalization.

   1. For generalization to other physical settings, the language instructor simply encounters the child in any setting other than where the language training occurred and presents him with the same visual and verbal stimuli.

   2. For generalization to other people, the language instructor instructs the classroom teacher, volunteer, peer or parent to present the same visual and verbal stimuli to the child and accurately report the response.

   3. For generalization to different discriminative stimuli, one must vary the visual and/or the verbal stimuli, while still requiring the same response.

   4. Generalization to similar tasks is more difficult to probe for until the child has a larger verbal repertoire to work with in that new words which utilize the same phonemes will probably have to be trained independently. However, the child should reach criterion in considerably fewer trials.

      Probes for similar task generalization are required as soon as the child can chain responses, e.g., "I want . . ." If the child has such a chain in his verbal repertoire, you can test his ability to generalize the use of this phrase by presenting him with a visual stimulus of any word in his repertoire and asking him, "What do you want? Say the whole thing."

B. *Generalization Training.* Select a minimum of two other people who will give the child the language training prescribed by the language instructor in at least two different settings. The only difference between this training and the training given by the language instructor is the number of trials required and, consequently, the amount of time involved. Only three or four trials on each specified task should be required. These can be presented to the child during storytime, math, lunch, etc., wherever it is agreeable for the person selected to do the generalization training. The language instructor must provide this person with cards which specify the discriminative stimuli, the criteria for a correct response, the reinforcement schedule and space to record the data [see Table 9-1]. These cards should be returned to the language instructor daily. When the child reaches criterion performance level with both generalization trainers in both settings, probing identical to that described above must be done to determine whether the child has generalized his language behaviors to other settings and people. (Murdock and Hartmann, in press, pp. 14-16).

Table 9-1 Generalization Training and Probing Cards

Child ________________

Date ________________

[Sample] Criteria for correct response:

1. Audible sound for every syllable.
2. "gl" blend may be "gw" in "glass."
3. "Wawa" is acceptable for "water."

[Sample] Desired response:

"I want a glass of water."

Setting / Trainer	Probe (S^D) Visual: Point to glass of water. Verbal: "What do you want? Say the whole thing."	Trials (R) Correct (+) Incorrect (-) Prompted Correct (p+) Prompted Incorrect (p-) No Response (0)				Reinforcement Schedule (S^R) and Tangible Reinforcer to be used

1. When probing: Do not reinforce, model, or prompt.
2. When training: Language instructor [therapist] will fill in the reinforcement schedule to be used as well as the tangible reinforcer.

   Language instructor will provide prompt to be used under S^D in addition to the verbal and visual stimuli.

   The generalization trainer should model the correct response immediately following any incorrect (-) response child makes, then present S^D again and record as usual.
3. Return these cards to language instructor daily so that data can be analyzed and appropriate cards set up for your next session. (Murdock and Hartmann, in press, p. 48).

TRANSFER THE PROGRAM TO CARETAKERS

The people who normally teach or rear the child are the natural ones to continue the modification effort after you leave. But you can't rely on a few hasty oral or written instructions to teach them how to do it. Nor can you provide them with a how-to-do-it book and leave them to their own devices. It might be helpful to ask a teacher or parent to read and master any one of a number of manuals on applications of behavior modification techniques in the classroom (e.g., Buckley and Walker, 1970; Homme et al., 1970; MacDonald, 1971; Sheppard, Shank, and Wilson, 1972) or in the home (e.g., Becker, 1971; Madsen and Madsen, 1972; Patterson and Gullion, 1968; Zifferblat, 1970). But this reading material should be viewed as an aid, not as the primary source for caretaker instruction. In a study of the comparative effectiveness of various methods for increasing the generalization and maintenance of child treatment effects, Walker and Buckley (1972) found that having teachers read a semiprogrammed behavior modification text and providing them some supervision and consultation was perhaps the least effective of the three methods used, although it was also the most time consuming. Providing the teachers with training and supervision in conducting the specific program previously used to increase the child's appropriate social and academic behavior proved much more effective in the maintenance of treatment gains. And this is the method we recommend.

While a number of effective parent- and teacher-training programs have been reported (see the reviews by Berkowitz and Graziano [1972] Johnson and Katz, [1973] and O'Dell [1974]), the procedures utilized have been very complex, typically including instruction in behavior principles and exposure to therapist models, in addition to cueing, verbal instruction and feedback regarding the caretakers' therapy attempts. This "shotgun" approach has made it difficult to identify the effective procedures with each program, so we are forced to continue to advocate complex training interventions, hoping that at least some of the component procedures will prove fruitful. We describe here a caretaker training program based largely on modeling and feedback techniques, and derived from our own experience (see Gelfand, Elton, and Harman, 1972).

Implementation

In your work with the child's caretakers, you will previously have explained to them the general outlines of the therapeutic procedure; the next step is to present them with a copy of the treatment script, and to invite them to observe you carry out a treatment session with their child. Immediately following the treatment session, make some arrangement for the child to absent himself (or, if you feel it would be helpful, include the child) and discuss the procedures in detail with the parents or teacher. If they seem confused or have difficulty following the sequence of procedures, it might be profitable to invite them to observe several more sessions. Then practice the treatment program with them. Let them take turns role-playing the therapist while you role-play the child. Let them rehearse until they feel comfortable with the procedures.

Next, help them carry out a treatment or training session with the child while you observe and cue them when necessary. The cueing can be accomplished by means of prearranged hand signals, gestures, or your holding up cardboard signs. If it would not be too disruptive, the easiest way to cue is simply to interrupt the proceedings and tell them what to do. If you have a standard audio tape recorder, a microphone (preferably one with an on-off switch), and a miniature earphone with a long extension cord, you can give the parent or teacher instructions as he carries out a session with the child (Stumphauzer, 1971). The adult trainee wears the earphone and you can transmit instructions to him via the microphone and tape recorder amplifier. The equipment needed, excluding the tape recorder and microphone, is available commercially for under $5, and enables you to train the caretakers by (a) making suggestions and prompts that will insure that their training attempts are successful, and (b) praising their good performance immediately after its occurrence.

The principles of behavior still obtain in this setting, so remember to praise the caretakers generously for their good or even slightly improved performances, but avoid appearing arrogant or condescending. They will naturally be sensitive about their inability to train their own child or pupil, and may be reluctant to accept instruction or advice on childbearing from a student who is himself just acquiring experience in child behavior modification.

Access to a tape recorder can further facilitate the process of parent or teacher training. An audio tape recorder (or, better yet, a video tape recorder) can be used to record the caretakers' therapy performances, and can be replayed for the purpose of analysis and feedback. You could record a training session that you conduct with the child and use this as a model for the procedure the caretaker should follow. Play the tape and discuss the procedure with him, advise him regarding problems he might encounter and offer suggestions in dealing with them. Then you could also tape one or more sessions conducted by the caretaker and later review the tape with him and discuss the good points as well as the flaws in his training performance. We have found such a video tape feedback instruction method to be helpful in teaching mothers and elderly volunteers to conduct standardized speech and imitation training sessions with young children enrolled in a day-treatment program (Gelfand et al., 1972). If at all possible, you should make yourself available for consultation, perhaps by telephone or correspondence, in case the caretakers later encounter difficulties in working independently.

PROGRAM PEER-GROUP SUPPORT FOR DESIRABLE BEHAVIOR

Busy teachers and parents often concentrate on other tasks to the near-complete exclusion of attending to and reinforcing the child's appropriate behavior (Hotchkiss, 1966; Madsen, Becker, and Thomas, 1968; Springmeyer, 1973). Consequently, the child's behavior may come more under the control of his classmates and siblings than of adults; and the other children may not influence his behavior in desirable ways. They may punish him a great deal (Ebner, 1967) with consequent ill effects, or may possibly urge him on to greater and greater feats of misbehavior. In fact, when playmates are pitted against adults as agents of control, the youngsters often prevail (Buehler, Patterson, and Furniss, 1966; Patterson, Cobb, and Ray, 1972). Further testimony to the power of the peer group is provided by the findings of Wolf, Hanley, King, Lachowicz, and Giles (1970) that a child's inappropriate out-of-seat activity in the classroom was more effectively controlled by his earning reinforcers for his entire class than if he alone earned reinforcers for remaining at his desk. Apparently, we neglect peer-group behavioral control at our own peril. Since it is not always possible to remove the child from a social group that fosters his misbehavior, it is sometimes necessary to redirect his peers' influence so that they stimulate and reinforce his prosocial activities. Consequently, if a therapist has not previously done so in the treatment program, he may wish to employ peers as change agents in the concluding phases of his intervention.

Examples

The preceding considerations led Patterson and his associates (Patterson, 1965; Patterson, Shaw, and Ebner, 1969; Ray, Shaw, and Cobb, 1970) to develop a signal device – a small box placed on the child's schoolroom desk, which could be operated to produce a light flash and a click. These events reinforced the child's studying, attending to the teacher, or otherwise complying with classroom regulations, and indicated that the child's efforts had earned points toward special privileges for the entire class. The use of signaling devices and group contingencies of this nature has rapidly brought children's disruptive behavior under control, and has proved to be a very effective means of promoting generalization and long-term maintenance of positive behavior change (Patterson et al., 1972; Walker and Buckley, 1972).

Walker and Buckley (1972) investigated various methods for increasing the scope and duration of treatment effects. These investigators first trained a child to work industriously at classroom assignments. Then group contingencies were applied to induce his classmates to encourage and support his work efforts. The research team made arrangements with each child's regular classroom teacher so that the child, through attending to his work and keeping his disruptive activities at a minimum, could earn the privilege of having the experimenter-therapists come to his classroom with their portable signaling unit. When the unit was present (during two, 30-minute periods scheduled twice a week), the child could earn points for himself and his classmates by his appropriate academic behavior; his inappropriate behavior lost points. Both points earned and points lost were signaled to the target child and his classmates. One of the other children recorded the points earned on a wall poster, and the target child was frequently applauded, cheered, and congratulated by the others for whom he had procured field trips, movies, parties, tickets to athletic events, and other reinforcers of their choice. This procedure was quite effective in maintaining treatment-produced increases in the target child's academic performance.

Implementation

A program such as Walker and Buckley's might be conducted even without special equipment. If you wished to do something like this, you would simply come to the child's classroom, observe his on-task versus off-task behavior, and record points earned and deducted on the schoolroom blackboard. In essence, the special apparatus is appealing, but probably not necessary to the procedure.

The number of points given and their buying power must be manipulated carefully so that the child can predictably perform well enough to earn the back-up reinforcers. The instructions given the child should emphasize the desirability of accumulating as many points as possible. For example, the Patterson group (Patterson et al., 1972, p. 13) set up contingencies specifying that "if the person chosen to play the game [the target child, of course] works real hard and gets 50 points, the whole class will get out five minutes early for recess today. If he works pretty hard and gets 30 points, the class gets out two minutes early." The child's work span is systematically extended by requiring him first to work or to attend for five seconds at a time and then, progressively, for ten seconds, 20 seconds, and up to a minute or more in order to earn points. For more information on sample schedules, see Ray et al. (1970).

The treatment manipulations just described presume that a therapist is available on a continuing basis to visit the school and award reinforcers. If the teacher can be taught to apply the same program, progress could take place even in the therapist's absence. Here, again, we need more research on training caretakers to act as therapeutic agents.

Probe Questions for Part 1, Chapter 9

1. Suppose that a therapist has successfully reduced a child's disruptive behavior in a reading class. The child no longer disrupts the reading class, but continues to act up during her arithmetic lessons. Was the therapy intervention a success? Why?

2. What are the potential problems associated with using a CRF schedule to shape and maintain a child's compliance with his parents' requests?

3. Give examples of naturalistic reinforcers and state why their use might be advisable.

4. As soon as Vanessa spies her therapist, she smiles, sits up straight, attends to the teacher, and does her schoolwork. When her therapist is not present, Vanessa stares out the window or whispers and giggles with nearby children. Why might the therapist's presence affect Vanessa's behavior in this way? How might the problem be remedied?

5. How might a child's peers be used to promote his desirable behaviors such as studying or (for a withdrawn child) speaking more frequently?

Behavioral Objectives for Part 2, Chapter 9

Studying this section should enable you to:

1. State the potential benefits derived from client self-regulation.

2. Help the child begin to monitor and regulate his own behavior.

3. Avoid the use of procedures that might antagonize the child or encourage his lying or cheating in self-regulation.

Part 2. Introducing Self-Regulation and Peer Control

It is possible to enhance the effectiveness and the durability of a treatment program by teaching the child to monitor and regulate his own behavior. While there is considerable current interest in the topic of self-regulation, and theoretical accounts of the process proliferate (Bandura, 1969; Kanfer and Phillips, 1970; Skinner, 1953; Thoresen and Mahoney, 1974), relatively few scientifically convincing clinical studies have appeared (Jeffrey, 1974) and even fewer of these deal with children. Nevertheless, several recent papers have indicated that children can accurately monitor and record their own performances and that these activities can have a beneficial impact on problem behaviors (Bolstad and Johnson, 1972; Broden, Hall, and Mitts, 1971). For example, Kaufman and O'Leary (1972) have found that adolescents enrolled in a token economy classroom in a psychiatric hospital program could maintain their decreased rates of disruptive behaviors during a one and one-half week self-evaluation period. First, reinforcement for cooperative behavior was administered systematically by the experimenters. When the adolescents' rates of disruptive activities had decreased appreciably, the self-evaluation procedure was introduced. During self-evaluation, each student was instructed to rate his own performance, to decide how many tokens he deserved, and to announce his decisions to his classmates and teacher. He then collected the number of tokens he had specified. Although the self-evaluative procedure was not imposed for an extended time period, and was not systematically varied to permit a thorough functional analysis, it was apparent that the students' improved classroom behavior was maintained during the self-evaluation phase of the experimental project.

Kaufman and O'Leary suggested that the self-evaluation procedure may have been effective for any of a number of reasons. For example, it is possible that the students found their new freedom reinforcing, that they feared that the program's failure would result in its discontinuation, that their improved study behaviors had become reinforcing, or that the back-up reinforcers acted to strengthen and maintain both self-evaluative statements and corresponding study behaviors. Whatever the reason, the student-conducted evaluation and contingency management resulted in much greater durability of desirable academic performance than does the abrupt withdrawal of tokens – a procedure that often produces a sudden, dramatic increase in students' disruptive behaviors. In view of these results, instruction in self-regulation may be worthwhile.

Warnings

The results of a recent study by Santogrossi, O'Leary, Romanczyk, and Kaufman (1973) indicate that self-evaluation training procedures are not invariably successful. This study is particularly valuable because it identifies some training procedures one should probably avoid. Santogrossi and his colleagues deserve commendation for their analysis of their program's probable inadequacies and for their suggestions to others who plan to instruct youngsters in self-regulation. Like Kaufman and O'Leary (1972), the Santogrossi group attempted to train adolescent psychiatric hospital patients in self-evaluation and self-reinforcement for appropriate study behavior. The latter project took place in an after-school remedial reading class. Following a training phase in which the teacher awarded the boys points exchangeable for snacks and prizes, the adolescents were allowed complete discretion in determining the points each had earned by nondisruptive behavior. Several of the boys quickly realized that they need not behave well in order to award themselves points. Their disruptive behavior reverted to baseline levels, and never thereafter returned to the low level first achieved under the teacher-determined point system. Furthermore, the boys became incensed at the subsequent introduction of a self-evaluation training system under which bonus points were awarded for accuracy and points deducted for inaccuracy of self-ratings. Because of the adolescents' extremely negative reaction and the threats of some of them to stop working at all, the matching system was discontinued after being in effect for only one day. Upon return to the teacher-determined point system, some reduction in their disruptive behavior took place, but when the completely self-determined point system was reintroduced, the boys' unruly behavior quickly returned to baseline levels.

Santogrossi and his colleagues attribute at least some portion of the treatment failure to inadequate length of training under the initial teacher-conducted token reinforcement system (nine days for this study as compared with 25 days in the successful Kaufman and O'Leary study). The duration of the externally administered reinforcement procedure may be an important factor. But Bolstad and Johnson (1972) obtained good results in a similar self-regulation program with disruptive first and second graders. Moreover, the teacher-conducted point system in the Bolstad and Johnson study lasted only six days. It may be important to include training in accuracy as a component of the initial instruction in self-evaluation. To be accurate, the child's evaluation of his own performance must correspond with an objective observer's evaluation of the child's performance. So, for instance, the child and the teacher must agree on the number of pages the child has read or the number of times he has disrupted the group. The Santogrossi Study did not require the adolescents to be accurate in their first attempts at self-evaluation. In contrast, Bolstad and Johnson incorporated accurate self-observation as a requirement for the children's receiving a maximal number of points in the first self-regulation phase of their experiment. Children whose self-observation ratings were within a range of three disruptive behaviors above or below an observer's score received the highest numbers of points, while those whose scores were less accurate received two less points than the observer's ratings indicated their behavior had merited. These accuracy requirements were not protested by the admittedly younger children treated by Bolstad and Johnson, and the youngsters successfully learned to assess and regulate their own classroom behavior. In view of these findings, therapists would be well advised to include accuracy training in self-evaluation instruction. Accuracy training seems far less likely to prove effective if introduced after the children have previously received unearned reinforcement for inaccuracy as occurred in the Santogrossi experiment.

The manner in which the self-regulation program is introduced to the children and the general circumstances surrounding the treatment should also be carefully planned. A program in any way imposed on children after school hours may be much less acceptable to them than similar training occurring during the course of their regular classroom instruction. The unsuccessful Santogrossi program was the only one of the three we have considered that took place after school hours. The additional schoolwork required may have irritated the boys and made them less willing to participate. They may well have viewed the extra academic effort demanded of them as an unwelcome intrusion into time they ordinarily spent in enjoyable recreational activities. Whatever the causes, the failure of this therapeutic effort indicates that transfer of control from teacher or therapist to the child himself must be handled with extreme care.

Implementation

Bandura (1969, Chapter 9; 1973, Chapter 5) offers a provocative account of how self-regulatory measures might be introduced into a treatment program for delinquent youths in order to produce a more extensive and lasting behavior change than is typically effected by institutional programs. It has been frequently observed that adolescents institutionalized for criminal offenses may behave impeccably while incarcerated, but revert to their typical antisocial activities immediately upon their release. Bandura argues that judicious environmental manipulation and training in contingency management can produce a more permanent positive impact on the delinquent adolescent's behavior. The same procedures might prove helpful in the treatment of other types of behavioral problems as well.

The therapist can serve as an exemplary model for the child, as Bandura points out. This indicates that you must yourself demonstrate the desired behavior patterns and standards for self-reinforcement. Don't have a temper tantrum and kick the wall or throw something while you are trying to teach the child self-control. You are being observed. Your conduct of the treatment program incidentally teaches the child how to regulate his own behavior (Grusec, 1966; Grusec and Mischel, 1966; Mischel and Grusec, 1966) and the behavior of others (Gelfand et al., 1974). Thus, if you reinforce the child's prosocial acts, he will become more likely to use similar reinforcement procedures when he serves as an instructor or supervisor.

Modeling procedures have played major roles in some treatment programs for juvenile offenders. In Sarason and Ganzer's (1969) project, youngsters were presented models of appropriate methods of dealing with everyday problems such as resisting peer appeals to engage in illegal activities, interacting with irritated supervisors, or responding nonviolently to other provocations. The delinquents were also given practice in role-playing appropriate reactions to common social conflict situations. Preliminary results indicated that modeling and guided practice programs of this nature improve both stated attitudes and social behavior of young offenders.

But the provision of exemplary models does not always suffice as an instructional device. It is often necessary to give specific, detailed training in self-assessment and contingency management as well. After the child's behavior has responded favorably to the contingencies imposed in the direct treatment program, an additional contingency can be imposed: that he must also accurately evaluate his own performance. A person who cannot reliably monitor and assess his own behavior probably cannot regulate it. Therefore, self-monitoring and evaluation are often considered necessary prerequisites for successful self-regulation (Kanfer and Phillips, 1970).

After the establishment of adequate self-assessment through giving differential reinforcement for accuracy, you must also train the child in the self-administration of reinforcers. He must learn to award himself reinforcers according to the same contingencies as were previously imposed on him by other people. Here, again, his adherence to the previously established external reinforcement contingency is itself reinforced. He gets an extra pay-off for reinforcing himself on schedule.

Since the ultimate goal is the production of an individual who can direct his own behavior appropriately, Bandura also recommends the gradual reduction of material rewards and an increasing reliance on less tangible self-administered, symbolic consequences such as a feeling of pride, a mental pat on the back, or telling a friend how well one is doing. While external environmental consequences beyond his control will continue to influence the person's behavior, he can himself manipulate his own experiences so that his desirable acts are consistently reinforced and his undesirable acts are not (Goldiamond, 1965; Homme, 1965; Skinner, 1953).

As Bandura suggests, the child or adolescent might also profit from instruction and practice in the application of contingency management programs to other children, particularly in the amelioration of behavior problems similar to his own. In the process, he will learn prosocial methods of behavioral control of others as well as of himself. In addition, this highly visible public commitment to and reinforcement of adherence to approved social codes might function to reverse the child's own attitudes concerning the desirability of theft, lying, of fist-fighting (Janis and King, 1954; Scott, 1957).

Finally, a change of social companions might be in order. If the child habitually associates with a group that values and reinforces antisocial behavior, one cannot expect him to remain a paragon of virtue. He must either change his associates or conform to their standards. In some cases, he must be taught new social skills, such as the art of carrying on a polite conversation with an adult, or the proper use of eating utensils, or how to express appreciation for a favor someone else has done for him. These new performances may be an important prerequisite for joining a more beneficial social group. A younger child might be taught athletic skills (how to catch, throw, and bat a softball, how to ride a bicycle) and personal hygiene habits (how and when to wash himself and brush his teeth) that could make him more acceptable to those classmates likely to have a positive impact on his social behavior. To summarize, the durability of behavioral improvements can be increased if you provide the child with appropriate models and associates, give him instruction in self-evaluation and contingency management, and somewhat decrease his reliance on external constraints. Additional techniques for training children in self-regulation are discussed in Part 5 of Chapter 5 on contingency contracting procedures.

Unfortunately, there are as yet few reliable guidelines on the establishment of self-regulatory functions. Table 9-2 presents several suggestions for self-regulation training that we have abstracted from the research data currently available. We will probably know more in the very near future, so watch professional journals such as the *Journal of Applied Behavior Analysis* and *Behavior Therapy* for the latest developments.

Table 9-2 Suggested Guidelines for Child Self-Regulation Training

DO make sure that the child is a willing partner in the self-regulation effort. His grudging participation will increase the likelihood of his cheating and the resulting failure of the program.

DO NOT impose the program on reluctant teenagers, particularly at times during which more attractive activities compete for their attention.

DO begin by applying to the child the same reinforcement contingency that you expect him to apply to himself later.

DO assess and reinforce the child's accuracy in self-evaluation.

If he proves inaccurate at first, DO use a shaping procedure to improve his accuracy of self-evaluation (as suggested by Santogrossi et al. [1973]).

DO NOT require the child to announce his self-evaluation to an antisocial peer group who might berate him for his foolishness at ever awarding himself less than the maximum possible number of points.

DO NOT threaten to fine him for inaccurate self-observations. (This coercive instruction enraged the adolescent delinquents in the Santogrossi study [1973]). DO phrase the instructions positively in terms of his accuracy as being well paid and inaccuracy as being less well paid.

DO fade artificial reinforcers from the program gradually while maintaining the child's self-regulation with occasional praise for his accomplishments.

Probe Questions for Part 2, Chapter 9

1. If you had the option of teaching any one of the following persons to apply the treatment program to the child, which one would you choose and why? (a) his mother, (b) his classmates, (c) the child himself.

2. Describe the methods one might use to control antisocial, delinquent behavior. Why is institutional treatment often ineffective?

3. State the conditions under which self-regulation training is likely to succeed or to fail.

4. In what ways might a child's companions increase his desirable behavior? How might they promote antisocial behavior?

Behavioral Objectives for Part 1, Chapter 10

After studying Part 1 of this chapter, you should be able to:

1. Summarize your reliability data and determine the degree of observer bias.

2. Determine whether your data require statistical analysis.

CHAPTER 10

Assessing the Effects of Your Treatment Program

Part 1. Summarizing Reliability Data and Determining Whether Your Data Require Statistical Analysis

By now you have completed the formal data gathering requirements of your study and terminated or reduced your therapeutic contacts with the child and his caretakers. While your regular data collection procedures have provided you with continuous measures of the progress of your study, it is now time to summarize those data systematically. It is the purpose of this chapter, then, to describe useful techniques for summarizing, analyzing, and presenting the data you have collected on the target behavior throughout the study. We will also describe for you the process of preparing a final report summarizing your project.

SUMMARIZING RELIABILITY DATA

The directions for summarizing your reliability data have been described in Part 2 of the chapter on reliability (Chapter 7). For your report, indicate the number of reliability check sessions, the phases during your study in which they were conducted, and the mean and range of your trial reliability estimates (see Table 7-6). If you used a multiple baseline design or more than two observers, these values should be reported for each target behavior and for each *pair* of observers. Should the observer totals reported in Table 7-6 prove to be discrepant, report the extent of the discrepancy and whether changes in the child's behavior were confounded with observer differences (see Chater 8, Part 2).

> Statistical evaluation of observer bias is accomplished by performing a *t*-test of the difference between correlated means on Observer 1's and 2's totals included in Table 7-6. The calculations required are described in elementary statistics texts.

IS A STATISTICAL ANALYSIS REQUIRED?

The usual (though not necessarily the best) method of analyzing sets of data in *N*=1 studies is a careful visual examination of the summarized data. For this reason, correct graphic methods are vitally important. Statistical analysis of *N*=1 data is also possible and necessary when the trends in the data are not obvious. While there are no firm rules for establishing whether a treatment effect is obvious from a visual inspection of the data, the paper by Freidman (1968) suggests a useful guideline based upon the amount of overlap

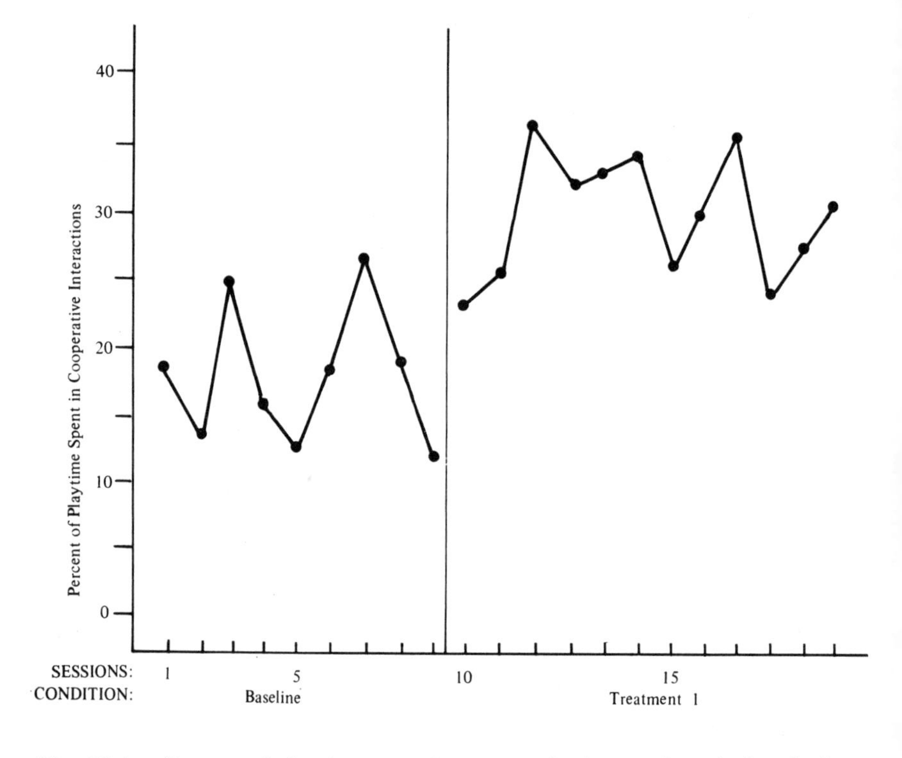

Fig. 10-1. Percent of playtime spent in cooperative interactions during the baseline and first treatment conditions.

of data points between treatment phases. This method assumes that we have at least five to ten data points in the baseline phase and a similar number of *stable* data points in each subsequent phase. By stable data points, we mean data points that show no consistent upward or downward trend. Thus, the data obtained at the beginning of a treatment or reversal condition would typically be excluded as the rate of the target behavior is (one hopes) increasing or decreasing at these times. If the data from two conditions are to be compared, construct a frequency distribution of the scores and determine the amount of overlap between the scores from the two conditions (i.e., the number of scores that appear in both conditions). If the percentage of overlapping scores is less than 50, it is probably not necessary to perform formal statistical analysis on the data from those two conditions.

We will illustrate this method with the data from Fig. 10-1. The first two data points in the treatment phase would be excluded from consideration as cooperative interactions are apparently increasing at this time. The frequency distribution of the remaining scores is shown in Fig. 10-2. Note that scores from the two conditions are identified by O's and X's. Examination of the degree of overlap of the data points from the two conditions suggests that

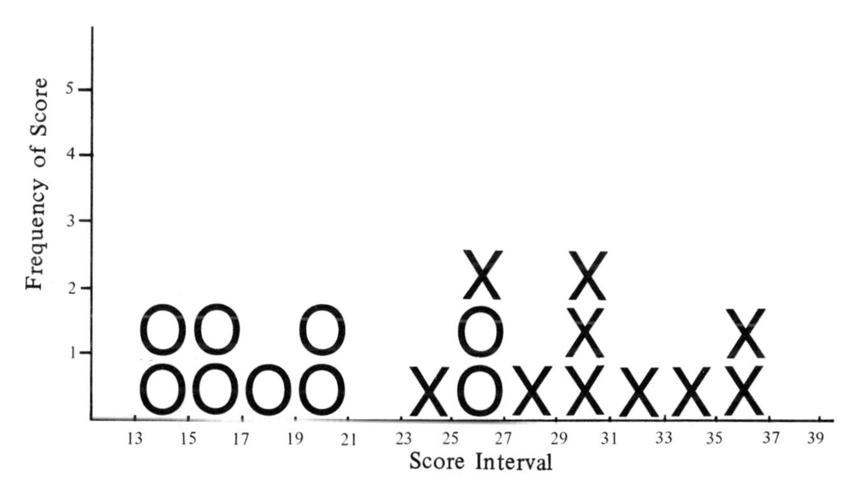

Fig. 10-2. Frequency distribution of percent of playtime spent in cooperative interactions during the baseline phase (O) and during Treatment 1 (x).

formal statistical analysis is unnecessary. Only four of the 19 scores (21%) overlap between the two conditions. Additional information on comparing data by simple graphs can be found in Darlington (1973).

Choosing the Appropriate Statistical Analysis

If the analysis of overlap suggests that formal statistical analysis is required, you have a number of alternative techniques to choose from depending upon the characteristics of the data, the number of conditions simultaneously being compared, and your own level of mathematical sophistication.

If it is only necessary to compare two sets of data at a time (e.g., treatment vs. baseline), and you have five to ten stable data points in each of the two conditions being compared, you might use either the Mann-Whitney *U* test or some other suitable nonparametric statistic (see Siegel, 1956). These tests are all well within the grasp of anyone who has completed an introductory statistics course.

For simultaneous comparisons involving more than two conditions (e.g., Baseline 1 and 2 and Treatment 1 and 2), other techniques are appropriate. If each condition to be compared contains ten to 12 stable data points (data that are not sequentially dependent), you might check one of the analysis of variance procedures suggested by Gentile, Roden, and Klein (1972) and Shine and Bower (1971). These procedures have a difficulty level of about intermediate statistics, and are generally adequate as long as the data subject to analysis are stable. If the data are not stable, serious mistakes in inference can be made with these procedures (see Hartmann, 1974, d).

Finally there is a class of procedures called time series analyses. These procedures are described by Gottman and his associates (Glass, Willson, and Gottman, 1973; Gottman, 1973; Gottman, McFall, and Barnett, 1969) and by Jones et al. (1973). While these techniques are ideally suited for N=1 data (as they do not presume stability), they do require substantial mathematical sophistication as well as the use of a computer.

If you think your data require statistical analysis, check with your instructor, and be sure to read carefully the material on choice of metric and averaging your data, which is included in Part 2 of this chapter.

Probe Questions for Part 1, Chapter 10

1. What reliability information should be included in your final report?

2. On what basis should the decision be made to omit formal statistical analysis of the target behavior?

3. What three classes of statistical analysis may be appropriate for N=1 data? Which one(s) can be used by someone with a modest degree of sophistication in statistics?

Behavioral Objectives for Part 2, Chapter 10

After studying Part 2 of this chapter, you should be able to:

1. Choose the best metric or form of your data for analysis (e.g., graphing).

2. State the factors that should be considered in determining how and when to group your data.

3. Determine the number of graphs necessary to clearly present your data.

4. Construct graphs of your data so that the results of your study can be easily understood.

Part 2. Summarizing and Graphing Target Behavior Data

GRAPHING YOUR DATA

Before constructing your final graphs, you must decide if and how the data should be averaged, how many graphs are needed to portray the data, and what form of the data should be used.

Choice of Metric

Depending on which form of data you choose to collect (see Chapter 3), you could represent your data either in terms of:
(a) absolute number (number of responses, intervals, or time),
(b) relative number (proportion of intervals or time), or
(c) rate per unit of time, such as hits per minute.

Although the three methods seem equally acceptable, there are many occasions when they are not; in fact, it is generally better to use either relative number or rate per unit of time rather than absolute number. Consider the case in which data collection periods vary in length from day to day, and the absolute number method is used. If the scores from irregular sessions were not prorated (see Part 1 of Chapter 8), daily "rate" changes might be interpreted as reflecting changes in the target behavior rather than as daily variation in the length of the observation period.

Another common example in which the absolute method might provide deceptive data is when the length of the generalization probes is consistently different (usually shorter) than the regular data collection session, and it is desirable to compare the data from the two sources. It may not be apparent, for example, that 27 responses in a seven-minute generalization probe is a rate different from 57 responses in a 20-minute regular data collection session. However, the rate of 3.86 responses per minute during the generalization probe would immediately be recognized as higher than 2.85 responses per minute during regular data collection.

In addition to making within-study comparisons easier, data expressed as rate per unit of time (either rate per minute for frequently occurring responses or rate per hour for infrequently occurring responses) also has the advantage of facilitating badly needed cross-study comparisons (Hartmann, 1972). Therefore, avoid the absolute method and use the rate per unit of time method if possible. For examples of data graphed in terms of rate per unit of time or proportion of time, see Figs. 10-5 and 10-6.

Averaging Your Data

Most, if not all, data are averaged over some period of time. The problem, then, is not usually whether to average but rather over what period of time to average the data. The most obvious answer to that question is to graph the data in daily session totals. Although minute-by-minute fluctuations within a session are lost by representing an entire session by a single number, these fluctuations are of little importance in evaluating your entire study (although they may be useful in suggesting variables that control the child's behavior).

At other times it may be useful to group your data over two, three, or even more sessions. If grouping over sessions seems desirable because of excessive variability in your data, the next question is how many session scores should be grouped. While this question has no simple answer, one major and a number of minor factors deserve consideration.

Fairness. The major factor you should consider is fairness – that is, to portray your data in a manner that fairly represents what actually occurred. The temptation is great to try a variety of different grouping procedures and then select the one that portrays the data in the most favorable light. This is not unlike the questionable practice of some group-design experimenters who try every conceivable statistical analysis on their data and then report the results of the particular analysis that are most favorable to the experimenter's favorite theory. Both the N=1 and group experimenter have exploited chance variations in their data and have obviously violated the fairness criterion.

The number of trials included in each session total. You should group the data if your target behavior has relatively few opportunities for occurrence each day, as would be the case for responses such as kissing mother when she returns from work or brushing teeth after each meal. Compare the ungrouped data portrayed in Fig. 10-3 with the grouped data portrayed in Fig. 10-4. In the former figure (the graph of daily occurrence-nonoccurrence of feeding the family pets) it is difficult to distinguish trends due to the treatment manipulation. When these same data are grouped over four-day sessions, the treatment effects are clear and easily distinguished (see Fig. 10-4).

The number of sessions included in each condition. Ordinarily, you will need more data collection sessions within each phase of your study if you group your data. For example, compare the treatment phase of Figs. 10-3 and 10-4 for the target behavior, feeding the dog. Before averaging over four-day periods (Fig. 10-3), this condition contained three data points; after averaging, it contained only a single data point. The latter case does not provide sufficient data to examine trends in the data across time.

If, early in your study, you are able to anticipate the number of sessions

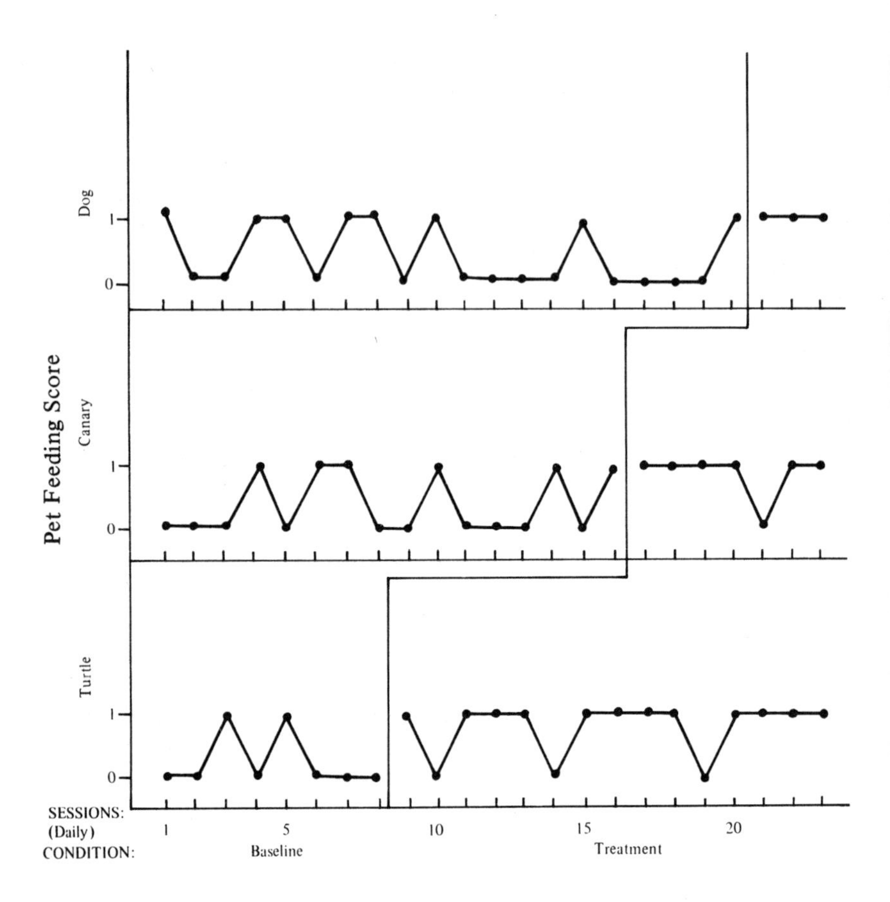

Fig. 10-3. Application of reinforcement procedures in a multiple baseline design to increase feeding of the family pets. Daily data are not collapsed.

over which your data will be grouped, try to use some multiple of that number for the number of sessions within each condition. For example, if you expect to group over four sessions, use eight, 12, or 16 sessions in each condition, so that you can avoid having to prorate your data.

If you are grouping data over, say, four-day intervals, and if the number of sessions in one or more conditions is not divisible by four, prorate your data. For example, if the totals for the three sessions of reversal were 14, 22, and 18, the average is 18 and the number you should graph is either 18, if you are plotting averages, or 72 (18 x 4), if you are plotting totals. Be sure to indicate in the figure legend when you have prorated your data.

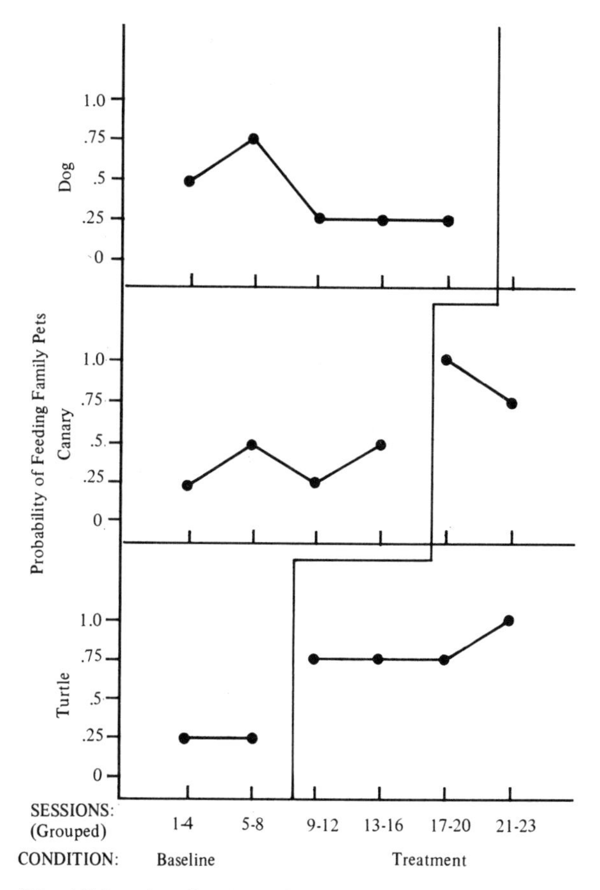

Fig. 10-4. Application of reinforcement procedures in a multiple baseline design to increase feeding of the family pets. Data are collapsed over four-day periods, except for the last data point for each behavior, which is based on three days of data.

Are your data cyclic? If your data indicate the presence of cyclic trends (see Fig. 8-1), it is generally advisable to group your data over the length of the cycle. That is, for four-day cycles, use a four-day grouping interval. The reason for this is simple: Your treatment effects, which have been superimposed on the cyclic trend, will be more easily discerned with the grouped data, as contrasted with the ungrouped data.

A final warning: If you group your data, be certain that you don't misrepresent them. The line between fudging your data and honestly representing them is sometimes a thin one, so take care that you don't fool your readers as well as yourself with misleading data manipulations.

If you think that grouping might in fact result in misrepresentation, you should include graphs of both the grouped and the ungrouped data. Readers can then reach their own conclusions.

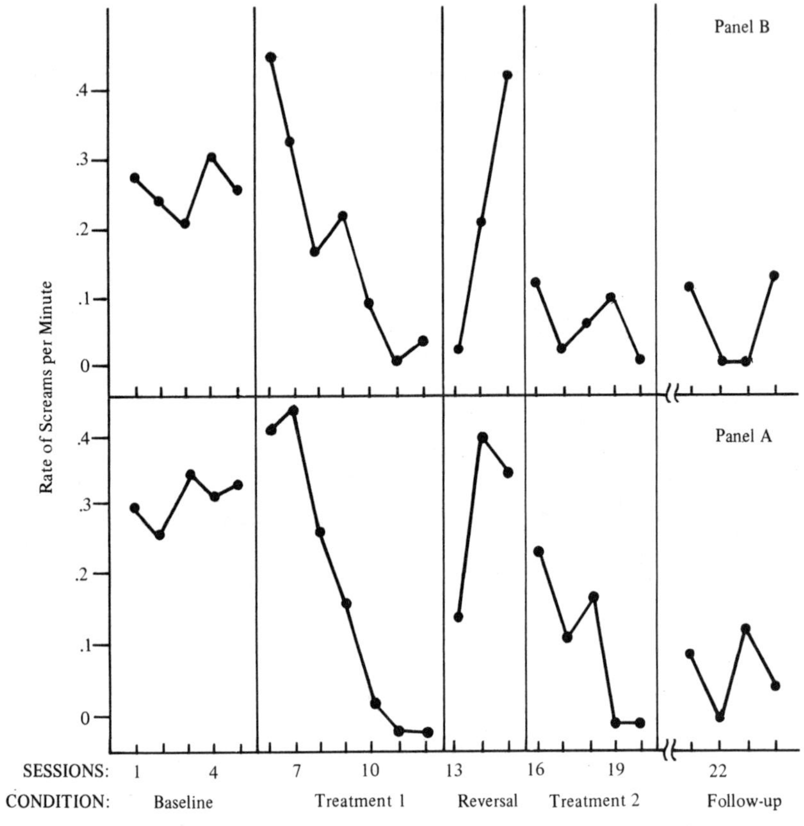

Fig. 10-5. Panel A shows the rate of the target behavior during regular data collection sessions. Panel B shows the rate of the target behavior during generalization probes. Follow-up began two weeks after the termination of treatment.

Number of Graphs

There are at least three situations when two or more graphs should be used to display your data. If you have used a multiple baseline design, it is generally best to use the "piggyback" format shown in Figs. 10-3 and 10-4.

You should also use this format if your treatment involved a combined acceleration-deceleration technique and you tabulated both the behavior to be increased and the behavior to be decreased. And, finally, use two or more graphs if you included generalization probes in your study and collected generalization data each day (or each day a training session was conducted). A sample graph of generalization data of this kind is presented in Fig. 10-5.

If you have included generalization probes only occasionally, indicate the generalization data on the same graph as is used for your regular data. Be sure, however, that both sources of data are expressed in the same rate measure and that a unique symbol is used for each source of data (see the example shown in Fig. 10-6).

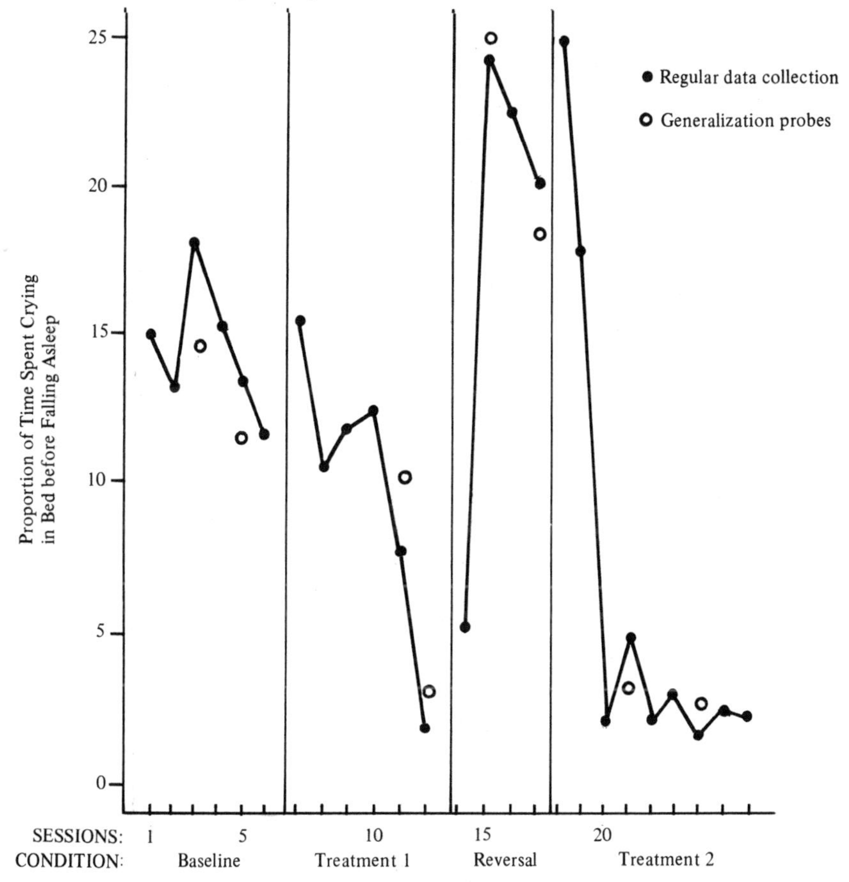

Fig. 10-6. Graph showing data from regular data collection sessions (afternoon nap) and periodic generalization probes (evening bedtime). (Note however for these data that it would have been preferable to begin treatment when the baseline was *not* descending.)

Constructing the Graphs

The graphs presented in this manual provide various models that may be relevant to your data. Additional information on graphing can be found in the American Psychological Association's *Publication Manual* (1974). When you construct the final graphs, be certain that they are neatly constructed and easy to interpret. To help you achieve this result, follow these rules:

1. Use a height-to-width ratio that is aesthetically pleasing; do not allow the graph itself to completely fill the page on which it occurs, as you must leave room for the figure legend, etc.

2. Clearly label both the horizontal and vertical axes. Begin the zero point about the horizontal baseline of the graph if you have zero entries. Failure to do so makes it difficult to discriminate the data line from the graph's horizontal baseline (compare Panel A of Fig. 10-7 with Panel B).

3. Use a vertical line to indicate conditions; break the line that connects the data points between conditions. Do not connect the first data point to zero on the vertical axis.

4. Use a curved hatched line to indicate breaks in the horizontal axis (see Fig. 10-5, horizontal axis of follow-up condition).

5. Make the data points sufficiently large so that they are not obliterated by the connecting line. (Compare Panel B of Fig. 10-7 with Panel A of the same figure.)

6. Prepare a figure legend that describes the content of the figure. This legend goes *below* the figure. If your graph needs qualifying – e.g., that some data points were prorated – indicate that in the figure legend. (The graph together with its legend should be understandable without reference to the text material.)

7. If you have more than one graph, number them consecutively.

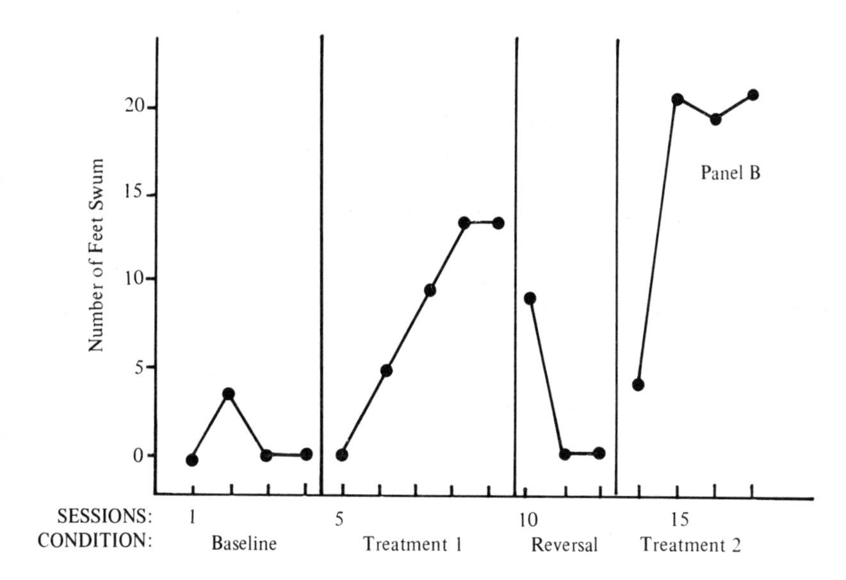

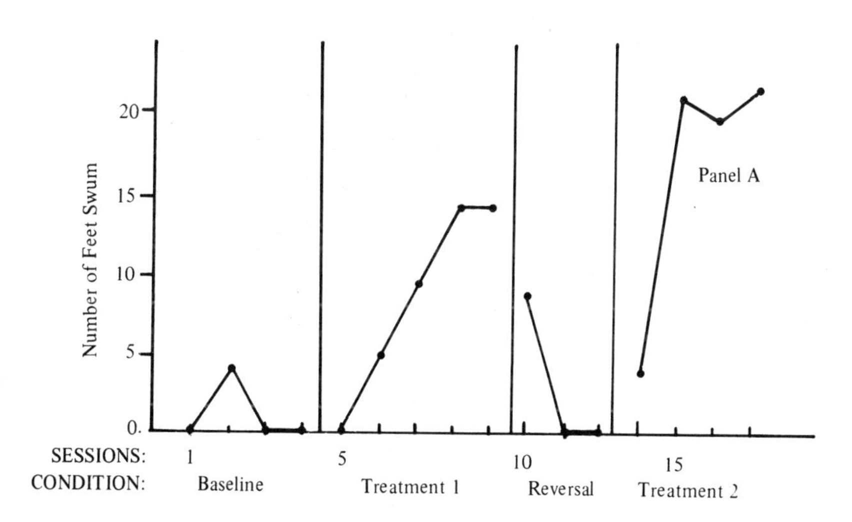

Fig. 10-7. Two graphs of the same data. In Panel A data points indicating zero rate lie on the ordinate; in Panel B data points indicating zero rate lie above the ordinate.

Probe Questions for Part 2, Chapter 10

1. What are the advantages and limitations of presenting data in terms of absolute number, relative number, and rate per unit of time?

2. How might an experimenter misrepresent his data by grouping them?

3. What factors should be given serious consideration when deciding whether to group and how to group data?

4. The figure given below violates many of the recommendations given in Part 2 of Chapter 10. How could the figure be improved?

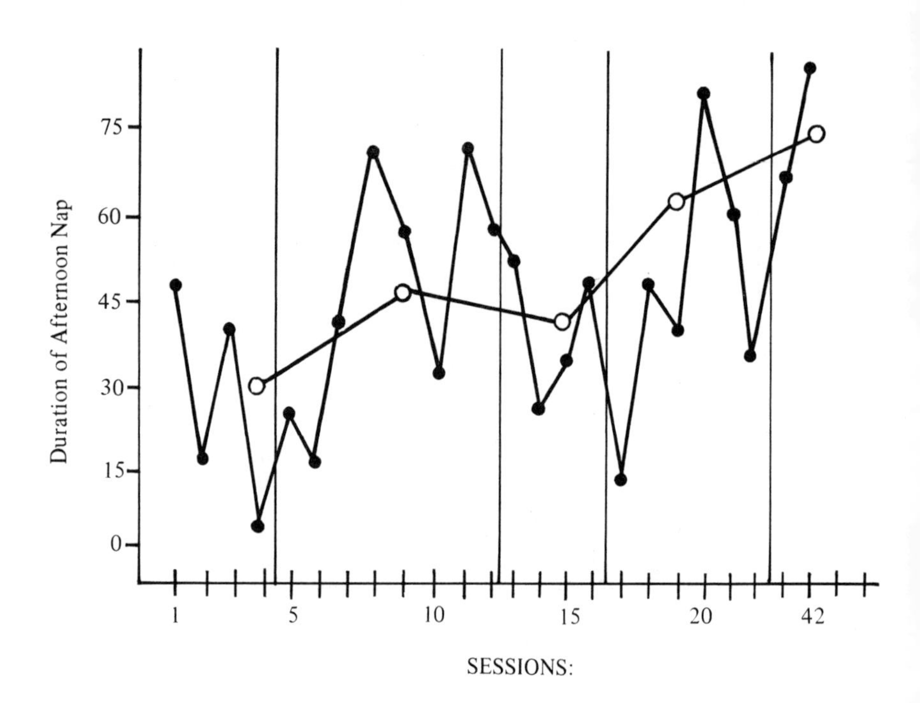

Behavioral Objectives for Part 3, Chapter 10

This section will help you to prepare a written report of your treatment project, and will offer suggestions for terminating your therapeutic relationships on a positive note.

Part 3. Writing a Final Report and Promoting Good Will

WRITING A REPORT

Now that you have collected, analyzed, and graphed the data on treatment-related changes in your child-client's behavior, you are ready to communicate your results to other people. You will want to do so with some detail and precision. Because it is preferable to have a permanent record of the behavior management program and its results, you will probably wish to write a final report. This report may meet an academic requirement or may simply be submitted as a courtesy to the school or agency in which your child-client is enrolled. Agency staff members or volunteers may decide to carry on the treatment effort you initiated. Therefore, a copy of your procedures, sample data sheets, and results and suggestions will prove helpful to them. This concluding section presents a format for use in preparing a final report and suggests some actions you might take to leave your clients and your instructor with a positive impression of your work.

The completed report should consist of the following sections:

1. Introduction, including an anecdotal description of the child-client and his behavioral deficits or excesses and a brief description of other published behavior modification programs dealing with the same target behavior.

2. A Method section precisely describing the target behavior, the goals of your treatment program, the experimental design used (e.g., a reversal or a multiple baseline design), and the treatment procedures you employed. Plans for collecting posttreatment follow-up data should also be explained.

3. A Results section, describing the reliability of your data and the method used to determine reliability. The Results section should also present the rates of the target behavior under baseline, treatment, and possibly under reversal and reintroduction of treatment program in the event you are using a reversal (ABAB) design. Any follow-up or generalization data available should also be reported.

4. Finally, a Discussion section summarizing the results obtained and the probable reasons for successes and failures, and suggested treatment program improvements. Table 10-1 illustrates the sequence and content of the various sections of a report.

If you have followed this manual's instructions faithfully, you will already have written a complete description of the target behavior and of the data recording procedures you used, as well as of the procedures followed during baseline, treatment, and reversal phases of the project. In addition, the methods of determining the quality of your data, including interobserver reliability, will have been described. This is nearly all the information you need for the Method section of your report. You will probably have completed one or more graphs displaying target behavior rates during all phases of the program, so a large part of your Results section is ready. You need only write a short Introduction, perhaps edit your Method section, describe the results as concisely as possible, discuss the merits and limitations of your program, and your report is completed. Published models for behavior modification treatment reports can be found in the *Journal of Applied Behavior Analysis* and *Behavior Therapy.*

Table 10-1 The Behavior Modification Program Report

I. *Introduction*
   A. Anecdotal description of the child (to protect his privacy, use a disguised name for the child in the report).
      1. Child's age and gender, general physical description.
      2. His family, siblings, the family's socioeconomic status, and anything remarkable about them or their situation (as long as this does not violate their anonymity).
      3. Child's reported behavior deficits or excesses.
      4. Who referred the child for help; their description of the problem.
      5. Previous attempts to modify this child's behavior and how they fared.
   B. Description of published behavior modification treatment programs dealing with the same or similar target behaviors. Cite each reference by author's last name and the date of publication – e.g. (Brown, 1969).
   C. Brief explanation of the intervention tactic employed and the reasons for using this rather than another technique – e.g., "Because Ben had never dressed himself, we devised a modification program for him which included modeling, verbal instructions, and shaping procedures."

II. *Method*
   A. The design used to demonstrate the effectiveness of the treatment program – e.g., "An ABAB reversal design was used; during the 'A' or baseline phases, Ernie's behavior was simply observed, while he received tokens for completing homework assignments during the treatment (B) phases."
   B. Precise and complete definitions of the target behavior, including behavioral descriptions of instances and of noninstances of target behavior.
   C. The recording and scoring procedures used. Include a sample data sheet.

D. Procedures followed in making baseline-phase behavior observations. This should include the setting, time of day, and weekly schedule of observation sessions. These should be the same as for treatment sessions.

E. Treatment procedures employed. This description should be sufficiently detailed to allow a reader to replicate your program. Include samples of training materials used if possible.

F. Plans for Future Treatment sessions or for collection of Follow-up data.

III. *Results*

A. Interobserver reliability values obtained. Describe how and when reliability checks were made. Explain reasons for low interobserver reliabilities, if necessary.

B. Analyses of observer effects. Explain, if necessary, how statements regarding treatment effectiveness must be qualified.

C. Respective rates of target performance during baseline and treatment phase of the program, and results of your data analysis. Present the data in graphic form and accompany them with a brief discussion of the rate changes observed. Also point out unusual circumstances, such as the child's being ill, that accompanied any remarkable rate fluctuations.

D. Follow-up or generalization data if available.

IV. *Discussion*

A. Summary of results obtained.

B. Probable reasons for the relative success or failure of the treatment program.

C. Suggestions for increasing the program's effectiveness.

D. Suggestions for caretakers. How can they maintain a child's improved behavior and teach him additional desirable behaviors. (Remember to offer only realistic advice; impractical solutions only discourage caretakers.)

E. Your plans, if any, for additional future work with this child.

V. *References*

Include here all the papers you have referred to in the body of your report. The most frequently used citation style used is that recommended by the American Psychological Association's *Publication Manual* (1974), and complete instructions for preparation of reference lists appear in that manual. A sample (fictitious) reference is as follows:

Brown, G.D. Treatment of a child's fear of dogs using an extinction procedure. *Journal of Experimental Child Behavior Analysis*, 1972, **43**, 101-113.

In this format the periodical's volume number is underlined to indicate italics, and the page numbers are presented last in the citation. The references are not numbered, and appear alphabetically by the first author's surname.

THANK YOU AND GOODBYE

When you converse with the persons involved in your program for the very last time, be sure that you give them a complete description of the results of the program (also supply them with your written report, if that is available) and that you express your appreciation for their cooperation. If the child is able to understand, you will probably want to explain the treatment results to him also and to show him the improvements he has made. As we pointed out initially, every treatment program involves costs as well as benefits, and the client and caretakers have borne some of those costs. Show them that you recognize this fact and are grateful. It is very important to treat school personnel and members of the community in such a way that they will be willing to work with your successors – the students who will conduct behavior modification projects in the future.

Just one more word on closing shop. Please be sure that any equipment you used is returned, is repaired if necessary, and is cleaned and ready for use by the next generation of students. Whether or not your department will remember you with pleasure will depend in part upon how you handled the program termination.

EPILOGUE

Now at last we come to the end of the lengthy process of child behavior therapy. If you have just completed your first such project, you will have realized that much additional supervised experience will be required before you can function independently as a professional therapist. You will have learned, perhaps to your surprise, that a great number and diversity of skills are necessary. The well-prepared therapist must have compassion and concern for his clients, must make sometimes painful and far-reaching decisions regarding the lives of others, and must acquire the human relations skills necessary to the success of any intervention program. The therapist must know the relevant state and federal statutes and regulations governing treatment, and must be aware of the ethical guidelines for his profession. In addition, the therapist must be a scholar – a reader of the therapy research literature, so that he can devise the most powerful treatment method available to help his client. He must be able to assess the problem accurately, observe reliably, and determine whether or not his treatment has had the desired effects. Furthermore, the therapist must upon occasion become a writer able to describe his procedures and results clearly for the instruction and information of readers. Humanist, scholar, practitioner, scientist, and writer – the behavior therapist must be all of these. We hope that this book has helped the reader progress at least a little way toward these ambitious goals.

Probe Questions for Part 3, Chapter 10

1. Describe the various sections of a written treatment program report and the information each section should contain.

2. What steps can you take to insure that the child, his teachers and family, and your sponsoring department will all remember you fondly?

Appendix A

INITIAL CARETAKER INTERVIEW

These are the basic questions to ask caretakers concerning the child's problem behavior:

1. *Specific Description.* Can you tell me what (child's name)'s problem seems to be?
   (If caretaker responds in generalities such as, "He is always grouchy," or that the child is rebellious, uncooperative, overly shy, then ask him to describe the behavior more explicitly.)
   What, exactly, does (he or she) do when (he or she) is acting this way?
   What kinds of things will (he or she) say?
2. *Last Incident.* Could you tell me just what happened the last time you saw (the child) acting like this?
   What did you do?
3. *Rate.* How often does this behavior occur?
   About how many times a day (or hour or week) does it occur?
4. *Changes in Rate.* Would you say this behavior is starting to happen more often, less often, or staying about the same?
5. *Setting.* In what situations does it occur?
   At home?
   At school?
   In public places or when (the child) is alone?
   (If in public places) Who is usually with him? How do they respond?
   At what times of day does this happen?
   What else is (the child) likely to be doing at the time?
6. *Antecedents.* What usually has happened right before (he or she) does this?
   Does anything in particular seem to start this behavior?
7. *Consequent Events.* What usually happens right afterward?
8. *Modification Attempts.* What things have you tried to stop (him or her) from behaving this way?
   How long did you try that?
   How well did it work?
   Have you ever tried anything else?

Appendix B

REINFORCER IDENTIFICATION LIST

Please indicate (child's name)'s favorite foods and activities on the checklist below. Make a checkmark opposite each item that is this child's particular favorite, then circle the three items you think he likes best of all.

1. *Foods*

______ brownies
______ cake: what kind(s)? ______________
______ candy: what kind(s)?______________
______ chewing gum: what brand(s)? ______________
______ cookies: what kind(s)? ______________
______ fruit: what kind(s)? ______________
______ nuts: what kind(s)? ______________
______ popcorn
______ popsicles: what flavor(s)? ______________
______ sugar-coated cereals: what brand(s)? ______________
______ other favorite foods (please specify) ______________________

____

2. *Drinks*

______ flavored milk: which flavor(s)? ______________
______ Koolaid: what flavor(s)?______________
______ milk
______ milkshakes: what flavor(s)? ______________
______ soft drinks: what kind(s)? ______________

Please indicate any foods or drinks this child is allergic to or any others he should not be given ____

____

3. *Playing Games and Sports*

boxing
______ camping
______ fishing
______ hide and seek
______ hiking
______ hopscotch
______ hunting

______ judo
______ jump rope
______ playground equipment (swings, climbing equipment, tether ball, seesaws) ________________ favorite(s)? ______________
______ playing baseball or softball
______ playing football
______ playing house
______ playing pool
______ playing in wading pool
______ riding in wagon
______ riding trike or bike
______ skiing
______ sledding or tubing
______ snorkeling
______ swimming
______ shooting basketballs
______ table tennis
______ tag
______ watching any of the above sports (please indicate which): ______

____

Does any physical illness or handicap prevent this child from full participation in sports or games? If so, please specify ______________________________

____

4. *Toys*

______ checkers
______ chess
______ constructing models: what kind(s)? ______________
______ construction toys (e.g., tinker toys, lego): what kind(s)? ________________
______ doing artwork: what kind(s)? ________________
______ playing board games or card games: what kind(s)? ______________
______ playing with cars or trucks
______ playing with dolls: what kind(s)? ________________
______ operating noise-making or moving toys: what kind(s)?____________
______ other favorite toys (please specify) ____________________

5. *Books*

______ books: favorite types? ____________________
______ comics: favorites? _____________________
______ magazines: favorites? ____________________
______ visit to library

6. *Opportunities to be with Others*

______ boys

  ____ younger ____ same age ____ older

______ girls

  ____ younger ____ same age ____ older

______ babies

______ adults

  ____ men ____ women

______ Boy or Girl Scouts, Campfire Girls

______ attending parties

______ holding parties

favorite companions ______________________________

7. *Play with or Care for Animals*

______ birds

______ cats

______ dogs

______ farm animals: what kind(s)? ________________

______ fish

______ horses

______ insects: what kind(s)? ________________

______ reptiles

______ turtles

8. *Travel*

______ amusement park

______ aviary

______ city parks

______ harbors

______ lakes and streams

______ mountains

______ museums and observatories

______ store

______ zoo

______ other local attractions: what kind(s)? e.g., dairies, mines

____

9. *Music and Dancing*

______ dancing: what kind(s)? ________________

______ phonograph records or tapes: favorites? ______________

______ playing a musical instrument: type(s)? ______________

______ singing: alone or with others? ______________

10. *Hobbies*

______ collecting: specify ______________

______ gardening

______ insect, bird, animal, plant identification (specify type)

____

______ other hobbies (specify) ______________________

11. ______ watching television: favorite programs? ______________

____

12. ______ attending movies: favorite types of films? ______________

____

13. ______ attending other types of meetings or performances: favorite types? ______________________

14. ______ having a room of one's own

______ being left alone, quiet

15. ______ helping mother, father, siblings around the house (circle the ones that apply)

______ playing with construction tools

______ playing with garden equipment

______ playing with mother's makeup

______ playing with pots and pans

Please remember to circle the three items this child likes best of all.

Thank you for your cooperation. This information will be most helpful in our constructing a program for this child.

References

Addison, R.M., and Homme, L. The reinforcing event (RE) menu. *NSPI Journal*, 1966, *V* (1), 8-9.

Alevizos, P.N., Campbell, M.D., Callahan, E.J., and Berck, P.L. Communication. *Journal of Applied Behavior Analysis,* 1974, **1**, 472.

Allen, K.E., Hart, B.M. Buell, J.S., Harris, F.R., and Wolf, M.M. Effects of social reinforcement on isolate behavior of a nursery school child. *Child Development,* 1964, **35**, 511-518.

American Association for Health, Physical Education, and Recreation. *How we do it game book: Selected games for the "How we do it" column of the Journal of Health-Physical Education-Recreation.* (3rd ed.) Washington, D.C.: American Association for Health, Physical Education, and Recreation, 1964.

American Psychological Association. *Ethical principles in the conduct of research with human participants.* Washington, D.C.: American Psychological Association, 1973.

American Psychological Association, Council of Editors. *Publication manual of the American Psychological Association.* (2nd ed.) Washington, D.C.: APA, 1974.

Anastasi, A. *Psychological testing.* (3rd ed.) New York: Macmillan, 1968.

Appel, J.B. Aversive aspects of a schedule of positive reinforcement. *Journal of the Experimental Analysis of Behavior,* 1963, **6**, 423-428.

Arnold, A. *Your child's play.* New York: Simon & Schuster, 1968.

Aronfreed, J., and Reber, A. Internalized behavioral suppression and the timing of social punishment. *Journal of Personality and Social Psychology,* 1965, **1**, 3-16.

Arrington, R.E. Time-sampling studies of child behavior. *Psychological Monographs,* 1939 **51**(2), 1-193.

Arrington, R.E. Time-sampling in studies of social behavior: A critical review of techniques and results with research suggestions. *Psychological Bulletin,* 1943, **60**, 81-124.

Association for Childhood Education International. *Equipment and supplies tested and approved for preschool, school, home.* Washington, D.C.: Association for Childhood Education International, 1964.

Atthowe, J.M., Jr., and Krasner, L. Preliminary report on the application of contingent reinforcement procedures: Token economy on a "chronic" psychiatric ward. *Journal of Abnormal Psychology,* 1968, **73**, 37-43.

Ayllon, T. Intensive treatment of psychotic behavior by stimulus satiation and food reinforcement. *Behaviour Research and Therapy,* 1963, **1**, 53-61.

Ayllon, T., and Azrin, N.H. Reinforcement and instructions with mental patients. *Journal of the Experimental Analysis of Behavior,* 1964, **7**, 327-331.

Ayllon, T., and Azrin, N.H. *The token economy: A motivational system for therapy and rehabilitation.* New York: Appleton-Century-Crofts, 1968.

Azrin, N.H. Effects of punishment intensity during variable-interval reinforcement. *Journal of the Experimental Analysis of Behavior*, 1960, **3**, 123-142.

Azrin, N.H. Time-out from positive reinforcement. *Science,* 1961, **133**, 383-384.

Azrin, N.H., and Holz, W.C. Punishment. In W. Honig (Ed.), *Operant behavior: Areas of research and application.* New York: Appleton-Century-Crofts, 1966. Pp. 380-447.

Baer, A.M., Rowbury, T., and Baer, D.M. The development of instructional control over classroom activities of deviant preschool children. *Journal of Applied Behavior Analysis,* 1973, **6**, 289-298.

Baer, D.M. Laboratory control of thumb sucking by withdrawal and representation of reinforcement. *Journal of the Experimental Analysis of Behavior,* 1962, **5**, 525-528.

Baer, D.M. Some remedial uses of the reinforcement contingency. In J.M. Shlien (Ed.), *Research in psychotherapy.* Vol. III. Washington, D.C.: American Psychological Association, 1968. Pp. 3-20.

Baer, D.M. A case for the selective reinforcement of punishment. In C. Neuringer and J.L. Michael (Eds.), *Behavior modification in clinical psychology.* New York: Appleton-Century-Crofts, 1970. Pp. 243-250.

Baer, D.M. Let's take another look at punishment. *Psychology Today,* 1971, **5**, 32-37.

Baer, D.M., and Wolf, M.M. The entry into natural communities of reinforcement. Paper presented at the meeting of the American Psychological Association, Washington, D.C., September 1967.

Baer, D.M., and Wolf, M.M. Recent examples of behavior modification in preschool settings. In C. Neuringer and J.L. Michael (Eds.), *Behavior modification in clinical psychology.* New York: Appleton-Century-Crofts, 1970. Pp. 10-25.

Baer, D.M., Wolf, M.M., and Risley,T.R. Some current dimensions of applied behavior analysis. *Journal of Applied Behavior Analysis*, 1968, **1**, 91-97.

Bailey, J.S., Timbers, G.D., Phillips, E.L., and Wolf, M.M. Modification of articulation errors of pre-delinquents by their peers. *Journal of Applied Behavior Analysis,* 1971, **4**, 265-281.

Bandura, A. Punishment revisited. *Journal of Consulting Psychology,* 1962, **26**, 298-301.

Bandura, A. *Principles of behavior modification.* New York: Holt, Rinehart and Winston, 1969.

Bandura, A. *Aggression: A social learning analysis.* Englewood Cliffs, N.J.: Prentice-Hall, 1973.

Bandura, A., Ross, D., and Ross, S.A. Imitation of film-mediated aggressive models. *Journal of Abnormal and Social Psychology,* 1963, **66**, 3-11.

Barron, F., and Leary, T. Changes in psychoneurotic patients with and without psychotherapy. *Journal of Consulting Psychology,* 1955, **19**, 239-245.

Barton, E.S. Inappropriate speech in a severely retarded child: A case study in language conditioning and generalization. *Journal of Applied Behavior Analysis,* 1970, **3**, 293-299.

Barton, E.S., Guess, D.G., Garcia, E., and Baer, D.M. Improvement of retardates' mealtime behaviors by time-out procedures using multiple baseline techniques. *Journal of Applied Behavior Analysis,* 1970, **3**, 77-84.

Becker, W.C. *Parents are teachers: A child management program.* Champaign, Ill.: Research Press, 1971.

Berkowitz, B.P., and Graziano, A.M. Training parents as behavior therapists: A review. *Behaviour Research and Therapy*, 1972, **10**, 297-318.

Bernal, M.E., Williams, D.E., Miller, W.H., and Reagor, P.A. The use of videotape feedback and operant learning principles in management of deviant children. In R. Rubin, H. Fensterheim, J. Henderson, and L. Ullmann (Eds.), *Advances in behavior therapy.* New York: Academic Press, 1972. Pp. 19-31.

Bijou, S.W., and Baer, D.M. *Child development: A systematic and empirical theory.* Vol. I. New York: Appleton-Century-Crofts, 1961.

Bijou, S.W., and Baer, D.M. Operant methods in child behavior and development. In W.K. Honig (Ed.), *Operant behavior: Areas of research and application.* New York: Appleton-Century-Crofts, 1966. Pp. 718-789.

Bijou, S.W., and Peterson, R.F. The psychological assessment of children: A functional analysis. In P. McReynolds (Ed.), *Advances in psychological assessment.* Vol. II. Palo Alto, Calif.: Science and Behavior Books, 1971. Pp. 63-78.

Bijou, S.W., Peterson, R.F., and Ault, M.H. A method to integrate descriptive and experimental field studies at the level of data and empirical concepts. *Journal of Applied Behavior Analysis*, 1968, **1**, 175-191.

Bijou, S.W., Peterson, R.F., Harris, F.R., Allen, K.E., and Johnston, M.S. Methodology for experimental studies of young children in natural settings. *Psychological Record,* 1969, **19**, 177-210.

Boer, A.P. Application of a simple recording system to the analysis of free-play behavior in autistic children. *Journal of Applied Behavior Analysis,* 1968, **1**, 335-340.

Bolstad, O.D., and Johnson, S.M. Self-regulation in the modification of disruptive classroom behavior. *Journal of Applied Behavior Analysis,* 1972, **5,** 443-454.

Boren, J.J., and Colman, A.D. Some experiments on reinforcement principles within a psychiatric ward for deliquent soldiers. *Journal of Applied Behavior Analysis,* 1970, **3,** 29-37.

Bostow, D.E., and Bailey, J.B. Modification of severe disruptive and aggressive behavior using brief time-out and reinforcement procedures. *Journal of the Experimental Analysis of Behavior,* 1969, **2,** 31-37.

Boyd, R.D., and DeVault, M.V. The observation and recording of behavior. *Review of Educational Research,* 1966, **36,** 529-551.

Broden, M. Notes on recording and on conducting a basic study. Unpublished manuscript, University of Kansas, undated.

Broden, M., Hall, R.V., and Mitts, B. The effect of self-recording on the classroom behavior of two eighth-grade students. *Journal of Applied Behavior Analysis*, 1971, **4**, 191-199.

Brown, P., and Elliott, R. Control of aggression in a nursery school class. *Journal of Experimental Child Psychology,* 1965, **2,** 103-107.

Bucher, B. Some ethical issues in the therapeutic use of punishment. In R. Rubin and C. Franks (Eds), *Advances in behavior therapy, 1968.* New York: Academic Press, 1969. Pp. 59-72.

Bucher, B. Some variables affecting children's compliance with instructions. *Journal of Experimental Child Psychology,* 1973, **15,** 10-21.

Bucher, B., and Lovaas, O.I. Use of aversive stimulation in behavior modification. In M.R. Jones (Ed.), *Miami symposium on the prediction of behavior: Aversive stimulation.* Coral Gables, Fla.: University of Miami Press, 1968. Pp. 77-145.

Buckley, N.K., and Walker, H.M. *Modifying classroom behavior: A manual of procedure for classroom teachers.* Champaign, Ill.: Research Press, 1970.

Buehler, R.E., Patterson, G.R., and Furniss, J.M. The reinforcement of behavior in institutional settings. *Behaviour Research and Therapy,* 1966, **4,** 157-167.

Buell, J., Stoddard, P., Harris, F., and Baer, D.M. Collateral social development accompanying reinforcement of outdoor play in a preschool child. *Journal of Applied Behavior Analysis*, 1968, **1**, 167-173.

Buist, C.A., and Schulman, J.L. *Toys and games for educationally handicapped children.* Springfield, Ill.: Thomas, 1969.

Burgess, R.L., Clark, R.N., and Hendee, J.C. An experimental analysis of anti-litter procedures. *Journal of Applied Behavior Analysis,* 1971, **4,** 71-75.

Campbell, B.A., and Church, R.M. *Punishment and aversive behavior.* New York: Appleton-Century-Crofts, 1969.

Campbell, D.T. Factors relevant to the validity of experiments in social settings. *Psychological Bulletin,* 1957, **54,** 297-312.

Campbell, D.T. The mutual methodological relevance of anthropology and psychology. In F. L. K. Hsu (Ed.), *Psychological anthropology.* Homewood, Ill.: Dorsey, 1961. Pp. 333-352.

Campbell, D.T., and Fiske, D. Convergent and discriminant validation by the multi-trait, multi-method matrix. *Psychological Bulletin,* 1959, **56,** 81-105.

Campbell, D.T., and Stanley, J.C. *Experimental and quasi-experimental designs for research.* Chicago: Rand McNally, 1963.

Cautela, J.R., and Kostenbaum, R. A reinforcement survey schedule for use in therapy, training, and research. *Psychological Reports,* 1967, **20,** 1115-1130.

Cheyne, J.A., and Walters, R.H. Intensity of punishment, timing of punishment, and cognitive structure as determinants of response inhibition. *Journal of Experimental Child Psychology,* 1969, **7,** 231-244.

Chittenden, G.E. An experimental study in measuring and modifying assertive behavior in young children. *Monographs of the Society for Research in Child Development,* 1942, **7** (1, Serial No. 31).

Christy, P.R. Does use of tangible rewards with individual children affect peer observers? Unpublished doctoral dissertation, University of Utah, 1973.

Christy, P.R., Gelfand, D.M., and Hartmann, D.P. Effects of competition-induced frustration on two classes of modeled behavior. *Developmental Psychology,* 1971, **5,** 104-111.

Church, R.M. The varied effects of punishment on behavior. *Psychological Review,* 1963, **70,** 369-402.

Cohen, J.A. A coefficient of agreement for nominal scales. *Educational and Psychological Measurement,* 1960, **20,** 37-46.

Cohen, J. Weighted Kappa: Nominal scale agreement with provision for scaled disagreement or partial credit. *Psychological Bulletin,* 1968, **70,** 213-220.

Cromer, C.C., Smith, C.L., Gelfand, D.M., Hartmann, D.P., and Page, B.C. The effects of instructional prompts and praise on children's altruistic behavior. Paper presented at the meeting of the Rocky Mountain Psychological Association, Denver, May 1974.

Cronbach, L.J. *Essentials of psychological testing.* (3rd ed.) New York: Harper & Row, 1970.

Cronbach, L.J., Gleser, G.C., Nanda, H., and Rajaratnam, N. *The dependability of behavioral measurements: Theory of generalizability for scores and profiles.* New York: Wiley, 1972.

D'Amato, M.R. *Experimental psychology: Methodology, psychophysics, and learning.* New York: McGraw-Hill, 1970.

Darlington, R.B. Comparing two groups by simple graphs. *Psychological Bulletin,* 1973, **79,** 110-116.

Davison, G.C., and Taffel, S.J. Effects of behavior therapy. Paper presented at the symposium on "Recent Evidence on the Effects of Divergent Therapeutic Methods," at the meeting of the American Psychological Association, Honolulu, September 1972.

Deese, J., and Hulse, S.H. *The psychology of learning.* New York: McGraw-Hill, 1967.

Donnelly, R.J., and Mitchell, E.D. *Active games and contests.* (2nd ed.) New York: Ronald Press, 1958.

Duncan, A.D. Self-application of behavior modification techniques by teenagers. *Adolescence,* 1969, **4,** 541-556.

Ebner, M. An investigation of the role of the social environment in the generalization and persistence of the effect of a behavior modification program. Unpublished doctoral dissertation, University of Oregon, 1967.

Edgington, E.S. *Statistical inference: The distribution-free approach.* New York: McGraw-Hill, 1969.

Etzel, B.C., and Gerwirtz, J.L. Experimental modification of caretaker-maintained high-rate operant crying in a 6 and a 20-week-old infant (*Infans Tyrannotearus*); Extinction of crying with reinforcement of eye contact and smiling. *Journal of Experimental Child Psychology,* 1967, **5,** 303-317.

Ferster, C.B., and Appel, J.B. Punishment of $S^{\triangle}$ responding in matching to sample by time-out from positive reinforcement. *Journal of the Experimental Analysis of Behavior,* 1961, **4,** 45-56.

Ferster, C.B., and Perrott, M.C. *Behavior principles.* New York: Appleton-Century-Crofts, 1968.

Ferster, C.B. and Skinner, B.F. *Schedules of reinforcement.* New York: Appleton-Century-Crofts, 1957

Fleiss, J.L. Measuring nominal scale agreement among many raters. *Psychological Bulletin,* 1971, **76,** 378-382.

Fleiss, J.L. *Statistical methods for rates and proportions.* New York: Wiley, 1973.

Fox, L. Effecting the use of efficient study habits. *Journal of Mathematics,* 1962, **1,** 75-86.

Foxx, R.M., and Azrin, N.H. The elimination of autistic self-stimulatory behavior by overcorrection. *Journal of Applied Behavior Analysis,* 1973, **6,** 1-14.

Franks, C.M., and Brady, J.P. Editorial: What is behavior therapy and why a new journal? *Behavior therapy,* 1970, **1,** 1-3.

Freidman, H. Magnitude of experimental effect and a table for its rapid estimation. *Psychological Bulletin,* 1968, **70,** 245-251.

Garcia, E., Baer, D.M., and Firestone, I. The development of generalized imitation within topographically determined boundaries. *Journal of Applied Behavior Analysis,* 1971, **4,** 101-112.

Gelfand, D.M. (Ed.) *Social learning in childhood: Readings in theory and application.* Belmont, Calif.: Brooks/Cole, 1969.

Gelfand, D.M., Elton, R.H., and Harman, R.E. A videotape-feedback training method to teach behavior modification skills to nonprofessionals. *Research in Education,* 1972, **7,** 15. (Abstract). Document ED 056 314, U.S. Office of Education.

Gelfand, D.M., and Hartmann, D.P. Behavior therapy with children. A review and evaluation of research methodology. *Psychological Bulletin,* 1968, **69,** 204-215.

Gelfand, D.M., Hartmann, D.P., Lamb, A.K., Smith, C.L., Mahan, M.A., and Paul, S.C. Effects of adult models and described alternatives on children's choice of behavior management techniques. *Child Development,* 1974, **45,** 585-593.

Gelfand, D.M., Hartmann, D.P., Smith, C.L., and Paul, S.C. The effects of adult models on children's choice of behavior management techniques. Paper presented at the annual meeting of the Rocky Mountain Psychological Association, Las Vegas, Nevada, May 1973.

Gellert, E. Systematic observation: A method in child study. *Harvard Educational Review,* 1955, **25,** 179-195.

Gentile, J.R., Roden, A.H., and Klein, R.D. An analysis-of-variance model for the intrasubject replication design. *Journal of Applied Behavior Analysis,* 1972, **5,** 193-198.

Glass, G.V., Willson, V.L., and Gottman, J.M. *Design and analysis of time-series experiments.* Boulder, Colo.: Laboratory of Educational Research, University of Colorado, 1973.

Goetz, E.M., and Baer, D.M. Social control of form diversity and the emergence of new forms in children's blockbuilding. *Journal of Applied Behavior Analysis,* 1973, **6,** 209-217.

Goldiamond, I. Self-control procedures in personal behavior problems. *Psychological Reports,* 1965, **17,** 851-868.

Goldstein, A.P., Heller, K., and Sechrest, L.B. *Psychotherapy and the psychology of behavior change.* New York: Wiley, 1966.

Goocher, B.E., and Ebner, M. A behavior modification approach utilizing sequential response targets in multiple settings. Paper presented at the meetings of the Midwestern Psychological Association, Chicago, May 1968.

Gottman, J.M. *N*-of-one and *N*-of-two research in psychotherapy. *Psychological Bulletin,* 1973, **80,** 93-105.

Gottman, J.M., McFall, R.M., and Barnett, J.T. Design and analysis of research using time series. *Psychological Bulletin,* 1969, **72,** 299-306.

Grusec, J. Some antecedents of self-criticism. *Journal of Personality and Social Psychology,* 1966, **4,** 244-252.

Grusec, J., and Mischel, W. Model's characteristics as determinants of social learning. *Journal of Personality and Social Psychology,* 1966, **4,** 211-214.

Guilford, J.P. *Fundamental statistics in psychology and education.* (4th ed.) New York: McGraw-Hill, 1965.

Hall, R.V., Cristler, C., Cranston, S.S., and Tucker, B. Teachers and parents as researchers using multiple baseline designs. *Journal of Applied Behavior Analysis,* 1970, **3,** 247-255.

Hall, R.V., Lund, D., and Jackson, D. Effects of teacher attention on study behavior. *Journal of Applied Behavior Analysis.* 1968, **1,** 1-12.

Harris, F.R., Johnston, M.K., Kelley, C.S., and Wolf, M.M. Effects of positive social reinforcement on regressed crawling of a nursery school child. *Journal of Educational Psychology,* 1964, **55,** 35-41.

Harris, F.R., Wolf, M.M., and Baer, D.M. Effects of adult social reinforcement on child behavior. *Young Children,* 1964, **20,** 8-17.

Hart, B.M., Allen, K.E., Buell, J.S., Harris, F.R., and Wolf, M.M. Effects of social reinforcement on operant crying. *Journal of Experimental Child Psychology,* 1964, **1,** 145-153.

Hart, B.M., and Risley, T.R. Establishing use of descriptive adjectives in the spontaneous speech of disadvantaged pre-school children. *Journal of Applied Behavior Analysis,* 1968, **1,** 109-120.

Hartley, R.E., and Goldenson, R.M. *The complete book of children's play.* New York: Crowell, 1963.

Hartmann, D.P. Techniques for evaluating research data. In D.M. Gelfand (Ed.), *Social learning in childhood.* Belmont, Calif.: Brooks/Cole, 1969. Pp. 1-14.

Hartmann, D.P. Some neglected issues in behavior modification with children. Paper presented at the sixth annual meeting of the American Association of Behavior Therapy, New York, October 1972.

Hartmann, D.P. Assessing the quality of observational data. Paper presented at the annual meeting of the Western Psychological Association, San Francisco, California, April 1974. (a)

Hartmann, D.P. A brief discussion of the stepwise criterion change design. Manuscript submitted for publication, 1974. (b)

Hartmann, D.P. Considerations in the choice of interobserver reliability estimates. Manuscript submitted for publication, 1974. (c)

Hartmann, D.P. Forcing square pegs into round holes: Some comments on "An analysis-of-variance model for the intrasubject replication design." *Journal of Applied Behavior Analysis*, 1974, **7,** 635-638. (d)

Hartmann, D.P., and Atkinson, C. Having your cake and eating it too! A note on some apparent contradictions between therapeutic achievements and design requirements in *N*=1 studies. *Behavior Therapy,* 1973, **4**, 589-591.

Hathaway, S.R. Some considerations relative to nondirective counseling as therapy. *Journal of Clinical Psychology*, 1948, **4**, 226-231.

Hauserman, N., Walen, S.R., and Behling, M. Reinforced racial integration in the first grade: a study in generalization. *Journal of Applied Behavior Analysis,* 1973, **6**, 193-200.

Hawkins, R.P., Peterson, R.F., Schweid, E., and Bijou, S.W. Behavior therapy in the home: Amelioration of problem parent-child relations with the parent in a therapeutic role. *Journal of Experimental Child Psychology,* 1966, **4**, 99-107.

Herbert, E.W. Response recording in the natural environment. Paper presented at the meeting of the California Behavior Modification Workshop, Stockton, Calif., May 1970.

Herbert, E.W. *Computation guide for interobserver reliabilities.* Salt Lake City: Bureau of Educational Research, University of Utah, 1973.

Herbert, E.W., Pinkston, E.M., Hayden, M.L., Sajwaj, T.E., Pinkston, S., Cordua, G., and Jackson, C. Adverse effects of differential parental attention. *Journal of Applied Behavior Analysis,* 1973, **6**, 15-30.

Herman, R.Z., and Azrin, N.H. Punishment by noise in an alternative response situation. *Journal of the Experimental Analysis of Behavior,* 1964, **7**, 185-188.

Herrickson, K., and Doughty, R. Decelerating undesired mealtime behavior in a group of profoundly retarded boys. *American Journal of Mental Deficiency,* 1967, **72**, 40-44.

Heyns, R.W., and Lippitt, R. Systematic observation techniques. In G. Lindzey (Ed.), *Handbook of social psychology.* Vol. 1. Reading, Mass.: Addison-Wesley, 1954. Pp. 370-404.

Hicks, D.J. Imitation and retention of film-mediated aggressive peer and adult models. *Journal of Personality and Social Psychology,* 1965, **2**, 97-100.

Holz, W.C., and Azrin, N.H. A comparison of several procedures for eliminating behavior. *Journal of the Experimental Analysis of Behavior,* 1963, **6**, 399-406.

Holz, W.C., Azrin, N.H., and Ayllon, T. Elimination of behavior of mental patients by response-produced extinction. *Journal of the Experimental Analysis of Behavior,* 1963, **6**, 407-412.

Homme, L.E. Perspectives in psychology – XXIV. Control of coverants: The operants of the mind. *Psychological Record,* 1965, **15**, 501-511.

Homme, L., Csanyi, A.P., Gonzales, M.A., and Rechs, J.R. *How to use contingency contracting in the classroom.* Champaign, Ill.: Research Press, 1970.

Homme, L.E., and Tosti, D.T. Contingency management and motivation. *National Society for Programmed Instruction Journal,* 1965, **4,** No.7.

Honigfeld, G. Non-specific factors in treatment: I. Review of placebo reactions and placebo reactors. *Diseases of the Nervous System,* 1964, **25,** 145-156.

Hopkins, B.L. Effects of candy and social reinforcements, instructions, and reinforcement schedule leaning on the modification and maintenance of smiling. *Journal of Applied Behavior Analysis,* 1968, **1,** 121-129.

Hopkins, B.L., Schutte, R.C., and Garton, K.L. The effects of access to a playroom on the rate and quality of printing and writing of first-and second-grade students. *Journal of Applied Behavior Analysis,* 1971, **4,** 77-87.

Hotchkiss, J.M. The modification of maladaptive behavior of a class of educationally handicapped children by operant conditioning techniques. Unpublished doctoral dissertation, University of Southern California, 1966.

Hutt, S.J., and Hutt, C. *Direct observation and measurement of behavior.* Springfield, Ill.: Thomas, 1970.

Jackson, D.A. A critical analysis of the multiple baseline design in applied behavior analysis. Unpublished manuscript, Department of Educational Research, University of Utah, Salt Lake City, Utah, 1973.

Jackson, D.A., Della-Piana, G.M., and Sloane, H.N., Jr. *Establishing a behavior observation system: a self instructional program.* Salt Lake City: Bureau of Educational Research, University of Utah, 1971.

Janis, I., and King, B. The influence of role playing on opinion change. *Journal of Abnormal and Social Psychology,* 1954, **49,** 211-218.

Jeffrey, D.B. Self-control: Methodological issues and research trends. In M.J. Mahoney and C.E. Thoresen (Eds), *Self-control: Power to the person.* Belmont, Calif.: Brooks/Cole, 1974. Pp. 166-199.

Jensen, A.R. The reliability of projective techniques: Methodology. *Acta Psychologica,* 1959, **16,** 108-136.

Johnson, C.A., and Katz, R.C. Using parents as change agents for their children: A review. *Journal of Child Psychology and Psychiatry,* 1973, **14,** 181-200.

Johnson, S.M., and Bolstad, O.D. Methodological issues in naturalistic observations: Some problems and solutions for field research. In L.A. Hamerlynck, L.C. Handy, and E.J. Mash (Eds.), *Behavior change: Methodology, concepts and practice. The fourth Banff international conference on behavior modification.* Champaign, Ill.: Research Press, 1973. Pp. 3-67.

Johnston, J.M. Punishment of human behavior. *American Psychologist,* 1972, **27,** 1033-1054.

Johnston, J.M., and Johnston, G.T. Modification of consonant speech-sound articulation in young children. *Journal of Applied Behavior Analysis,* 1972, **5,** 233-246.

Johnston, M.K., and Harris, F.R. Observation and recording of verbal behavior in remedial speech work. In H. Sloan and B. MacAulay (Eds.), *Operant procedures in remedial speech and language training.* New York: Houghton-Mifflin, 1968. Pp. 40-60.

Johnston, M.K., Kelley, C.S., Harris, F.R., Wolf, M.M., and Baer, D.M. Effects of positive social reinforcement on isolate behavior of a nursery school child. Unpublished manuscript, University of Washington, 1964.

Jones, R.R. Design and analysis problems in program evaluation. In P.O. Davidson, F.W. Clark, and L.A. Hamerlynck (Eds.), *Evaluation of behavioral programs in community, residential, and school settings.* Champaign, Ill.: Research Press, 1974. Pp. 1-31.

Jones, R.R., Vaught, R.S., and Reid, J.B. Time series analysis as a substitute for single analysis of variance designs. Paper presented at the Symposium on "Methodological Issues in Applied Behavior Analysis," at the meetings of the American Psychological Association, Montreal, Quebec, Canada, September 1973.

Kanfer, F.H. Issues and ethics in behavior manipulation. *Psychological Reports,* 1965, **16**, 187-196.

Kanfer, F.H., and Phillips, J.S. *Learning foundations of behavior therapy.* New York: Wiley, 1970.

Kanfer, F.H., and Saslow, G. Behavioral analysis: An alternative to diagnostic classification. *Archives of General Psychiatry,* 1965, **12**, 529-538.

Kanfer, F.H., and Saslow, G. Behavioral diagnosis. In C.M. Franks (Ed.), *Behavior therapy: Appraisal and status.* New York: McGraw-Hill, 1969. Pp. 417-444.

Kantor, J.R. *Interbehavioral psychology.* Bloomington: Principia Press, 1958.

Katz, R.C. Interactions between the facilitative and inhibitory effects of a punishing stimulus in the control of children's hitting behavior. *Child Development,* 1971, **42**, 1433-1446.

Kaufman, K.F., and O'Leary, K.D. Reward, cost, and self-evaluation procedures for disruptive adolescents in a psychiatric hospital school. *Journal of Applied Behavior Analysis,* 1972, **5**, 293-310.

Kazdin, A.E. Response cost: The removal of conditioned reinforcers for therapeutic change. *Behavior Therapy,* 1972, **3**, 533-546.

Kazdin, A.E., and Bootzin, R.R. The token economy: An evaluative review. *Journal of Applied Behavior Analysis,* 1972, **5**, 343-372.

Keller, F.S. A personal course in psychology. In R. Ulrich, T. Stachnik, and J. Mabry (Eds.), *The control of behavior.* Glenview, Ill.: Scott, Foresman, 1966. Pp. 91-93.

Keller, F.S. "Good-bye-teacher . . ." *Journal of Applied Behavior Analysis,* 1968, **1**,79-89.

Kerlinger, F.N. *Foundations of behavioral research.* New York: Holt, Rinehart and Winston, 1964.

Kimble, G.A. *Hilgard and Marquis' conditioning and learning.* (2nd ed.) New York: Appleton-Century-Crofts, 1961.

Kirby, F.D., and Toler, H.C., Jr. Modification of preschool isolate behavior: A case study. *Journal of Applied Behavior Analysis,* 1970, **3**, 309-314.

Koegel, R.L., and Rincover, A. Treatment of psychotic children in a classroom environment: I. Learning in a large group. Unpublished manuscript, University of California, Los Angeles, 1973.

Krasner, L. Behavior control and social responsibility. *American Psychologist,* 1964, **17**, 199-204.

Krasner, L. Behavior therapy. In P.H. Mussen and M.R. Rosenzweig (Eds.), *Annual review of psychology.* Vol. 22. Palo Alto, Calif.: Annual Reviews, 1971. Pp. 483-532.

Krasner, L., and Krasner, M. Token economies and other planned environments. In C.E. Thoresen (Ed.), *Behavior modification 1973, the seventy-second yearbook of the National Society for the Study of Education.* Chicago: University of Chicago Press, 1973. Pp. 351-381.

Kraus, R.G. *Play activities for boys and girls six through twelve: A guide for teachers, parents, and recreation leaders.* New York: McGraw-Hill, 1957.

Krippendorff, K. Bivariate agreement coefficients for reliability of data. In E.F. Borgatta and G.W. Bohrnstedt (Eds.), *Sociological Methodology 1970.* San Francisco: Jossey-Bass, 1970. Pp. 139-150.

Lahey, B.B. Modification of the frequency of descriptive adjectives in the speech of Head Start children through modeling without reinforcement. *Journal of Applied Behavior Analysis,* 1971, **4**, 19-22.

Lamb, A.K.M. Effects of response alternatives, success and failure, and model competence on children's imitation of adult's score-keeping behavior. Unpublished master's thesis, University of Utah, 1973.

Lana, R.E. Pre-test sensitization. In R. Rosenthal and R.L. Rosnow (Eds.), *Artifact in behavioral research.* New York: Academic Press, 1969. Pp. 121-146.

Latchaw, M. *Pocket guide of games and rhythms for the elementary school.* Englewood Cliffs, N.J.: Prentice-Hall, 1970.

Leitenberg, H. Is time-out from positive reinforcement an aversive event? A review of the experimental evidence. *Psychological Bulletin,* 1965, **64**, *428-44*

Lepper, M.R., Greene, D., and Nisbett, R.E. Undermining children's intrinsic interest with extrinsic reward: A test of the "overjustification" hypothesis. *Journal of Personality and Social Psychology,* 1973, **28**, 129-137.

Lovaas, O.I. Behavior therapy approach to treatment of childhood schizophrenia. In J.P. Hill (Ed.), *Minnesota symposium on child development.* Vol. 1. Minneapolis: University of Minnesota Press, 1967. Pp. 108-159.

Lovaas, O.I., Freitag, G., Gold, V.J., and Kassorla, I.C. Recording apparatus and procedure for observation of behaviors of children in free play settings. *Journal of Experimental Child Psychology,* 1965, **2**, 108-120.

Lovaas, O.I., and Simmons, J.Q. Manipulation of self-destruction in three retarded children. *Journal of Applied Behavior Analysis*, 1969, **2**, 143-157.

MacDonald, W.S. *Battle in the classroom: Innovations in classroom techniques.* Scranton, Pa.: Intext Educational Publishers, 1971.

Madsen, C.H., Jr., Becker, W.C., and Thomas, D.R. Rules, praise, and ignoring: Elements of elementary classroom control. *Journal of Applied Behavior Analysis,* 1968, **1**, 139-150.

Madsen, C.H., Jr., Becker, W.C., Thomas, D.R., Koser, L., and Plager, E. An analysis of the reinforcing function of "Sit-down" commands. In R.K. Parker (Ed.), *Readings in educational psychology.* Boston: Allyn & Bacon, 1968. Pp. 265-278.

Madsen, C.K., and Madsen, C.H., Jr. *Parents/children/discipline: A positive approach.* Boston: Allyn & Bacon, 1972.

Maloney, K.B., and Hopkins, B.L. The modification of sentence structure and its relationship to subjective judgement of creativity in writing. *Journal of Applied Behavior Analysis*, 1973, **6**, 425-433.

Marks, I.M., and Gelder, M.G. Transvestism and fetishism: Clinical and psychological changes during faradic stimulation. *British Journal of Psychiatry,* 1967, **113,** 711-729.

Martin, M.F., Gelfand, D.M., and Hartmann, D.P. Effects of adult and peer observers on boys' and girls' responses to an aggressive model. *Child Development,* 1971, **42,** 1271-1275.

McMillan, D.E. A comparison of the punishing effects of response-produced shock and response-produced time-out. *Journal of the Experimental Analysis of Behavior,* 1967, **10,** 430-449.

McNamara, J.R., and MacDonough, T.S. Some methodological considerations in the design and implementation of behavior therapy research. *Behavior Therapy,* 1972, **3**, 361-379.

McReynolds, L.V. Application of time-out from positive reinforcement for increasing the efficiency of speech training. *Journal of Applied Behavior Analysis,* 1969, **2**, 199-207.

Medley, D.M., and Mitzel, H.E. Measuring classroom behavior by systematic observation. In N.L. Gage (Ed.), *Handbook of research on teaching.* Chicago: Rand McNally, 1963. Pp. 247-328.

Meichenbaum, D.H., Bowers, K., and Ross, R.R. Modification of classroom behavior of institutionalized female adolescent offenders. *Behaviour Research and Therapy,* 1968, **6**, 343-353.

Merton, R.K. *Social theory and social structure.* New York: Free Press, 1968.

Millenson, J.R. *Principles of behavioral analysis.* New York: Macmillan, 1967.

Minge, M.R., and Ball, T.S. Teaching of self-help skills to profoundly retarded patients. *American Journal of Mental Deficiency,* 1967, **71**, 864-868.

Mischel, W. *Personality and assessment.* New York: Wiley, 1968.

Mischel, W., and Grusec, J. Determinants of the rehearsal and transmission of neutral and aversive behaviors. *Journal of Personality and Social Psychology,* 1966, **3**, 197-205.

Murdock, J.Y., and Hartmann, B. *A language development program: Imitative gestures to basic syntactic structures.* Salt Lake City: Word Making Productions, in press.

Neale, J.M., and Liebert, R.M. *Science and behavior: An introduction to methods of research.* Englewood Cliffs, N.J.: Prentice-Hall,1973.

Nelson, J.D., Gelfand, D.M., and Hartmann, D.P. Children's aggression following competition and exposure to aggressive models. *Child Development,* 1969, **40**, 1085-1097.

Neuringer, C., and Michael, J.L. *Behavior modification in clinical psychology.* New York: Appleton-Century-Crofts, 1970.

Nunnally, J. *Psychometric theory.* New York: McGraw-Hill, 1967.

O'Brien, F., and Azrin, N.H. Developing proper mealtime behaviors of the institutionalized retarded. *Journal of Applied Behavior Analysis,* 1972, **5**, 389-399.

O'Brien, F., Azrin, N.H., and Bugle, C. Training profoundly retarded children to stop crawling. *Journal of Applied Behavior Analysis,* 1972, **5**, 131-137.

O'Brien, F., Bugle, C., and Azrin, N.H. Training and maintaining a retarded child's proper eating. *Journal of Applied Behavior Analysis,* 1972, **5**, 67-72.

O'Connor, R.D. Modification of social withdrawal through symbolic modeling. *Journal of Applied Behavior Analysis,* 1969, **2**, 15-22.

O'Dell, S. Training parents in behavior modification: A review. *Psychological Bulletin,* 1974, **81**, 418-433.

O'Leary, K.D. Behavior modification in the classroom: A rejoinder to Winett and Winkler. *Journal of Applied Behavior Analysis,* 1972, **5**, 505-510.

O'Leary, K.D., Becker, W.C., Evans, M.B., and Saudargas, R.A. A token reinforcement program in a public school: A replication and systematic analysis. *Journal of Applied Behavior Analysis,* 1969, **2**, 3-13.

O'Leary, K.D., and Drabman, R. Token reinforcement programs in the classroom: A review. *Psychological Bulletin,* 1971, **75**, 379-398.

O'Leary, K.D., and Kent, R. Behavior modification for social action: Research tactics and problems. In L.A. Hamerlynck, L.C. Handy, and E.J. Mash (Eds.), *Behavior change: Methodology, concepts and practice. The fourth Banff international conference on behavior modification.* Champaign, Ill.: Research Press, 1973. Pp. 69-118.

O'Leary, K.D., Poulos, R.W., and Devine, V.T. Tangible reinforcers: Bonuses or bribes? *Journal of Consulting and Clinical Psychology,* 1972, **38**, 1-8.

Orne, M.T. On the social psychology of the psychological experiment: With special reference to demand characteristics and their implications. *American Psychologist,* 1962, **17**, 776-783.

Parke, R.D. Effectiveness of punishment as an interaction of intensity, timing, agent nurturance and cognitive structuring. *Child Development,* 1969, **40**, 213-235.

Parke, R.D. The role of punishment in the socialization process. In R. Hoppe, G. Milton, and E. Simmel (Eds.), *Early experiences and the process of socialization.* New York: Academic Press, 1970. Pp. 81-107.

Patterson, G.R. An application of conditioning techniques to the control of a hyperactive child. In L.P. Ullmann and L. Krasner (Eds.), *Case studies in behavior modification.* New York: Holt, Rinehart and Winston, 1965. Pp. 370-375.

Patterson, G.R., Cobb, J.A., and Ray, R.S. Direct intervention in the classroom: A set of procedures for the aggressive child. In F.W. Clark, D.R. Evans, and L.A. Hamerlynck (Eds.), *Implementing behavioral programs in educational and clinical settings.* Champaign, Ill.: Research Press, 1972. Pp. 151-201.

Patterson, G.R., and Gullion, M.E. *Living with children.* Champaign, Ill.: Research Press, 1968.

Patterson, G.R., and Harris, A. Some methodological considerations for observation procedures. Paper presented at the meetings of the American Psychological Association, San Francisco, September 1968.

Patterson, G.R., McNeal, S., Hawkins, N., and Phelps, R. Reprogramming the social environment. *Journal of Child Psychology and Psychiatry,* 1967, **8**, 181-195.

Patterson, G.R., Ray, R.S., Shaw, D.A., and Cobb, J.A. *Manual for coding family interactions,* 1969. Available from ASIS National Auxillary Publication Service, care of CMM Information Sciences, Inc., 909 3rd Ave., New York, N.Y. 10022. Document #01234.

Patterson, G.R., Shaw, D.A., and Ebner, M.J. Teachers, peers, and parents as agents of change in the classroom. In F.A.M. Benson (Ed.), *Modifying deviant social behaviors in various classroom settings.* Eugene, Ore.: University of Oregon Press, 1969. Pp. 13-47.

Paul, G.L. Behavior modification research: Design and tactics. In C.M. Franks (Ed.), *Behavior therapy: Appraisal and status.* New York: McGraw-Hill, 1969. Pp. 29-62.

Pawlicki, R. Behaviour-therapy research with children: A critical review. *Canadian Journal of Behavioural Science/Revue Canadienne Des Sciences Du Comportement,* 1970, **2**, 163-173.

Peterson, D.R. *The clinical study of social behavior.* New York: Appleton-Century-Crofts, 1968.

Phillips, E.L. Achievement Place: Token reinforcement procedures in a home-style rehabilitation setting for "pre-delinquent" boys. *Journal of Applied Behavior Analysis,* 1968, **1**, 213-223.

Phillips, E.L., Phillips, E.A., Fixsen, D.L., and Wolf, M.M. Achievement Place: Modification of the behaviors of pre-delinquent boys within a token economy. *Journal of Applied Behavior Analysis,* 1971, **4**, 45-59.

Premack, D. Toward empirical behavior laws: I. Positive reinforcement. *Psychological Review,* 1959, **66**, 219-233.

Ray, R.S., Shaw, D.A., and Cobb, J.A. The work box: An innovation in teaching attentional behavior. *The School Counselor,* 1970, **18**, 15-35.

Reese, H.W., and Parnes, S.J. Programming creative behavior. *Child Development,* 1970, **41**, 413-423.

Reid, J.B. Reliability assessment of observation data: A possible methodological problem. *Child Development,* 1970, **41**, 1143-1150.

Revusky, S.H. Some statistical treatments compatible with individual organism methodology. *Journal of the Experimental Analysis of Behavior,* 1967, **10**, 319-330.

Reynolds, N.J., and Risley, T.R. The role of social and material reinforcers in increasing talking of a disadvantaged preschool child. *Journal of Applied Behavior Analysis*, 1968, **1**, 253-262.

Risley, T.R. The effects and side effects of punishing the autistic behaviors of a deviant child. *Journal of Applied Behavior Analysis,* 1968, **1**, 21-34.

Risley, T.R. Behavior modification: An experimental-therapeutic endeavor. In L.A. Hamerlynck, P.O. Davidson, and L.E. Acker (Eds.), *Behavior modification and ideal mental health services.* Calgary: University of Calgary Press, 1969. Pp. 103-127.

Risley, T.R., and Baer, D.M. Operant behavior modification: The deliberate development of behavior. In B. Caldwell and H. Ricciuti (Eds.), *Review of child development research: Social influence and social action.* Vol. III. Chicago: University of Chicago Press, 1973. Pp. 283-329.

Risley, T.R., and Wolf, M.M. Strategies for analyzing behavior change over time. In J.R. Nesselroade and H.W. Reese (Eds.), *Lifespan developmental psychology: Methodological issues.* New York: Academic Press, 1973. Pp. 175-183.

Ritter, B. The group treatment of children's snake phobias using vicarious and contact desensitization procedures. *Behaviour Research and Therapy,* 1968, **6**, 1-6.

Roethlisberger, F.J., and Dickson, W.J. *Management and the worker.* Cambridge, Mass.: Harvard University Press, 1939.

Rogers, C.R., and Skinner, B.F. Some issues concerning the control of human behavior: A symposium. *Science,* 1956, **124**, 1057-1066.

Rosenthal, D., and Frank, J.D. Psychotherapy and the placebo effect. *Psychological Bulletin,* 1956, **53,** 294-302.

Rosenthal, R. *Experimenter effects in behavior research.* New York: Appleton-Century-Crofts, 1966.

Rosenthal, R., and Rosnow, R.L. *Artifact in behavior research.* New York: Academic Press, 1969.

Ross, A.O. *Psychological disorders of children.* New York: McGraw-Hill, 1974.

Sajwaj, T., Twardosz, S., and Burke, M. Side effects of extinction procedures in a remedial preschool. *Journal of Applied Behavior Analysis,* 1972, **5,** 163-175.

Salzberg, B.H., Wheeler, A.J., Devar, L.T., and Hopkins, B.L. The effect of intermittent feedback and intermittent contingent access to play on printing of kindergarten children. *Journal of Applied Behavior Analysis,* 1971, **4,** 163-171.

Santogrossi, D.A., O'Leary, K.D., Romanczyk, R.G., and Kaufman, K.F. Self-evaluation by adolescents in a psychiatric hospital school token program. *Journal of Applied Behavior Analysis,* 1973, **6,** 277-287.

Sarason, I.G., and Ganzer, V.J. Social influence techniques in clinical and community psychology. In C.D. Spielberger (Ed.), *Current topics in clinical and community psychology.* Vol. 1. New York: Academic Press, 1969. Pp. 1-66.

Schaeffer, H.H., and Martin, P.L. *Behavioral therapy.* New York: McGraw-Hill, 1969.

Schumaker, J., and Sherman, J.A. Training generative verb usage by imitation and reinforcement procedures. *Journal of Applied Behavior Analysis,* 1970, **3,** 273-287.

Schutte, R.C., and Hopkins, B.L. The effects of teacher attention on following instructions in a kindergarten class. *Journal of Applied Behavior Analysis,* 1970, **3,** 117-122.

Schwitzgebel, R.L., and Schwitzgebel, R.K. (Eds.) *Psychotechnology: Electronic control of mind and behavior.* New York: Holt, 1973.

Scott, W.A. Attitude change through reward of verbal behavior. *Journal of Abnormal and Social Psychology,* 1957, **55,** 72-75.

Sears, R.R., Maccoby, E.E., and Levin, H. *Patterns of child rearing.* Evanston: Row, Peterson, 1957.

Sheppard, W.C., Shank, S.B., and Wilson, D. *How to be a good teacher: Training social behavior in young children.* Champaign, Ill.: Research Press, 1972.

Shine, L.C., II, and Bower, S.M. A one-way analysis of variance for single-subject designs. *Educational and Psychological Measurement,* 1971, **31,** 105-113.

Sidman, M. *Tactics of scientific research.* New York: Basic Books, 1960.

Siegel, S. *Nonparametric statistics.* New York: McGraw-Hill, 1956.

Skiba, E.A., Pettigrew, L.E., and Alden, S.E. A behavioral approach to the control of thumbsucking in the classroom. *Journal of Applied Behavior Analysis,* 1971, **4,** 121-125.

Skinner, B.F. *Science and human behavior.* New York: Macmillan, 1953.

Skinner, B.F. *Verbal behavior.* New York: Appleton-Century-Crofts, 1957.

Skinner, B.F. What is the experimental analysis of behavior? *Journal of the Experimental Analysis of Behavior,* 1966, **9,** 213-218.

Sloane, H.N., Jr., and MacAulay, B.D. *Operant procedures in remedial speech and language training.* Boston: Houghton Mifflin, 1968.

Solomon, R.L. Punishment. *American Psychologist,* 1964, **19,** 239-253.

Springmeyer, L.B. Stimulus variation transition from behavior modification treatment to regular classroom. Unpublished doctoral dissertation, University of Utah, 1973.

Stuart, R.B. Behavioral contracting within the families of delinquents. *Journal of Behavior Therapy and Experimental Psychiatry,* 1971, **2,** 1-11.

Stumphauzer, J.S. A low-cost "bug-in-the-ear" sound system for modification of therapist, parent, and patient behavior. *Behavior Therapy,* 1971, **2,** 249-250.

Swenson, E.W. The effect of instruction and reinforcement on the behavior of geriatric psychiatric patients. Unpublished doctoral dissertation, University of Utah, 1965.

Tate, B.G., and Baroff, G.S. Aversive control of self-injurious behavior in a psychotic boy. *Behaviour Research and Therapy*, 1966, **4,** 281-287.

Terrace, H.S. Discrimination learning with and without "errors." *Journal of the Experimental Analysis of Behavior,* 1963, **6,** 1-27.

Terrace, H.S. Stimulus control. In W. Honig (Ed.), *Operant behavior: Areas of research and application.* New York: Appleton-Century-Crofts, 1966. Pp. 271-344.

Tharp, R.G., and Wetzel, R.J. *Behavior modification in the natural environment.* New York: Academic Press, 1969.

Thomas, J.R. Avoidance of time-out from two VI schedules of positive reinforcement. *Journal of the Experimental Analysis of Behavior,* 1964, **7,** 168.

Thompson, D.M. Escape from $S^{\triangle}$ associated with fixed-ratio reinforcement. *Journal of the Experimental Analysis of Behavior*, 1964, **7,** 1-8.

Thoresen, C.E., and Mahoney, M.J. *Behavioral self-control.* New York: Holt, Rinehart and Winston, 1974.

Tukey, J.W. *Exploratory data analysis.* Reading, Mass.: Addison-Wesley, 1970.

Twardosz, S., and Sajwaj, T. Multiple effects of a procedure to increase sitting in a hyperactive retarded boy. *Journal of Applied Behavior Analysis,* 1972, **5,** 73-78.

Tyler, V.O., and Brown, D.G. The use of swift, brief isolation as a group control device for institutionalized delinquents. *Behaviour Research and Therapy,* 1967, **5**, 1-9.

Ullmann, L.P. On cognitions and behavior therapy. *Behavior Therapy,* 1970, **1**, 201-204.

Ulrich, R.E., and Azrin, N.H. Reflexive fighting in responses to aversive stimulation. *Journal of the Experimental Analysis of Behavior,* 1962, **5**, 511-520.

Underwood, B.J. *Psychological research.* New York: Appleton-Century-Crofts, 1957.

Wahler, R.G. Oppositional children: A quest for reinforcement control. *Journal of Applied Behavior Analysis,* 1969, **2**, 159-170.

Wahler, R.G., Winkel, G.H. Peterson, R.F., and Morrison, D.C. Mothers as behavior therapists for their own children. *Behaviour Research and Therapy,* 1965, **3**, 113-124.

Walker, H.M., and Buckley, N.K. The use of positive reinforcement in conditioning attending behavior. *Journal of Applied Behavior Analysis,* 1968, **1**, 245-250.

Walker, H.M., and Buckley, N.K. Programming generalization and maintenance of treatment effects across time and across settings. *Journal of Applied Behavior Analysis,* 1972, **5**, 209-224.

Walker, H.M., and Buckley, N.K. *Token reinforcement techniques.* Eugene, Oregon: E-B Press, 1974.

Walker, H.M., Mattson, R.H., and Buckley, N.K. The functional analysis of behavior within an experimental class setting. In W.C. Becker (Ed.), *An empirical basis for change in education.* Chicago: Science Research Associates, 1971. Pp. 236-263.

Walters, R.H., and Parke, R.D. The influence of punishment and related disciplinary techniques on the social behavior of children: Theory and empirical findings. In B.A. Maher (Ed.), *Progress in experimental personality research.* Vol. 4. New York: Academic Press, 1967. Pp. 179-228.

Webb, E.J., Campbell, D.T., Schwartz, R.D., and Sechrest, L. *Unobtrusive measures: Nonreactive research in the social sciences.* Chicago: Rand McNally, 1966.

Weick, K.E. Systematic observational methods. In G. Lindzey and E. Aronson (Eds.), *The handbook of social psychology.* (2nd ed.) Menlo Park, Calif.: Addison-Wesley, 1968. Pp. 357-451.

Weiner, H. Some effects of response cost upon human operant behavior. *Journal of the Experimental Analysis of Behavior,* 1962, **5**, 201-208.

Welsh, R.S. The use of stimulus satiation in the elimination of juvenile firesetting behavior. In A.M. Graziano (Ed.), *Behavior therapy with children.* Chicago: Aldine-Atherton, 1971. Pp. 283-289.

Wexler, D.B. Token and taboo: Behavior modification, token economies, and the law. *California Law Review,* 1973, **61**, 81-109.

Whaley, D.L., and Malott, R. *Elementary principles of behavior.* New York: Appleton-Century-Crofts, 1971.

Whelan, P. Reliability of human observers. Unpublished doctoral dissertation, University of Utah, Salt Lake City, Utah, June 1974.

White, G.D., Nielsen, G., and Johnson, S.M. Timeout duration and the suppression of deviant behavior in children. *Journal of Applied Behavior Analysis,* 1972, **5**, 111-120.

Whitman, T.L., Zakaras, M., and Chardos, S. Effects of reinforcement and guidance procedures on instruction-following behavior of severely retarded children. *Journal of Applied Behavior Analysis,* 1971, **4**, 283-290.

Wiggins, J.S. *Personality and prediction: Principles of personality assessment.* Reading, Mass.: Addison-Wesley, 1973.

Williams, C.D. The elimination of tantrum behavior by extinction procedures. *Journal of Abnormal and Social Psychology,* 1959, **59**, 269.

Winer, B.J. *Statistical principles in experimental design.* (2nd ed.) New York: McGraw-Hill, 1971.

Winett, R.A., and Winkler, R.C. Current behavior modification in the classroom: Be still, be quiet, be docile. *Journal of Applied Behavior Analysis,* 1972, **5**, 499-504.

Wolf, M.M., Birnbrauer, J.S., Williams, T., and Lawler, J. A note on the apparent extinction of vomiting behavior of a retarded child. In L.P. Ullmann and L. Krasner (Eds.), *Case studies in behavior modification.* New York: Holt, Rinehart and Winston, 1965. Pp. 364-365.

Wolf, M., Hanley, E., King, L., Lachowicz, J., and Giles, D. The timer-game: A variable interval contingency for the management of out-of-seat behavior. *Exceptional Children,* 1970, **37**, 113-118.

Wolf, M.M., Phillips, E.L., and Fixsen, D.L. The teaching family: A new model for the treatment of deviant child behavior in the community. In S.W. Bijou and E.L. Ribes (Eds), *Behavior modification: Issues and extensions.* New York: Academic Press, 1972. Pp. 51-62.

Wolf, M.M., and Risley, T.R. Reinforcement: Applied research. In R. Glaser (Ed.), *The nature of reinforcement.* New York: Academic Press, 1971. Pp. 310-325.

Wolf, M.M., Risley, R.T., Johnston, M., Harris, F., and Allen, E. Applications of operant conditioning procedures to the behavior problems of an autistic child: A follow-up and extension. *Behaviour Research and Therapy,* 1967, **5**, *103-111.*

Wolf, M.M., Risley, T.R., and Mees, H.L. Application of operant conditioning procedures to the behavior problems of an autistic child. *Behaviour Research and Therapy,* 1964, **1**, 305-312.

Wolpe, J. *The practice of behavior therapy,* (2nd ed.) New York: Pergamon Press, 1973.

Worthy, R.C. A miniature, portable timer and audible signal-generating device. *Journal of Applied Behavior Analysis,* 1968, **1**, 159-160.

Wright, H.F. Observational child study. In P.H. Mussen (Ed.), *Handbook of research methods in child development.* New York: Wiley, 1960. Pp. 71-139.

Wright, H.F. *Recording and analyzing child behavior.* New York: Harper & Row, 1967.

Zeilberger, J., Sampen, S., and Sloane, H. Modification of a child's problem behavior in the home with the mother as therapist. *Journal of Applied Behavior Analysis,* 1968, **1**, 47-53.

Zifferblat, S.M. *You can help your child improve study and homework behaviors.* Champaign, Ill.: Research Press, 1970.

Zimmerman, E.H., Zimmerman, J., and Russel, C.D. Differential effects of token reinforcement on instruction-following behavior in retarded students as a group. *Journal of Applied Behavior Analysis,* 1969, **2**, 101-112.

Zimmerman, J., and Baydan, N.T. Punishment of $S^{\triangle}$ responding of humans in conditional matching to sample by timeout. *Journal of the Experimental Analysis of Behavior,* 1963, **4**, 589-597.

Zimmerman, J., and Ferster, C.B. Intermittent punishment of $S^{\triangle}$ responding in matching to sample. *Journal of the Experimental Analysis of Behavior,* 1963, **3**, 349-356.

Zimmerman, J., and Ferster, C.B. Some notes on time-out from positive reinforcement. *Journal of the Experimental analysis of Behavior,* 1964, **7**, 13-19.

Zlutnick, S.I. The control of seizures by the modification of preseizure behavior: The punishment of behavioral chain components. Unpublished doctoral dissertation, University of Utah, 1972.

Author Index

Subject Index

TITLES IN THE PERGAMON GENERAL PSYCHOLOGY SERIES

Vol. 1. J. WOLPE–*The Practice of Behavior Therapy, Second Edition*
Vol. 2. T. MAGOON *et al.*–*Mental Health Counselors at Work*
Vol. 3. J. McDANIEL–*Physical Disability and Human Behavior, Second Edition*
Vol. 4. M.L. KAPLAN *et al.*–*The Structural Approach in Psychological Testing*
Vol. 5. H.M. LaFAUCI & P.E. RICHTER–*Team Teaching at the College Level*
Vol. 6. H.B. PEPINSKY *et al.*–*People and Information*
Vol. 7. A.W. SIEGMAN & B. POPE–*Studies in Dyadic Communication*
Vol. 8. R.E. JOHNSON–*Existential Man: The Challenge of Psychotherapy*
Vol. 9. C.W. TAYLOR–*Climate for Creativity*
Vol. 10. H.C. RICKARD–*Behavioral Intervention in Human Problems*
Vol. 11. P. EKMAN, W.V. FRIESEN & P. ELLSWORTH–*Emotion in the Human Face: Guidelines for Research and an Integration of Findings*
Vol. 12. B. MAUSNER & E.S. PLATT–*Smoking: A Behavioral Analysis*
Vol. 14. A. GOLDSTEIN–*Psychotherapeutic Attraction*
Vol. 15. F. HALPERN–*Survival: Black/White*
Vol. 16. K. SALZINGER & R.S. FELDMAN–*Studies in Verbal Behavior: An Empirical Approach*
Vol. 17. H.E. ADAMS & W.K. BOARDMAN–*Advances in Experimental Clinical Psychology*
Vol. 18. R.C. ZILLER–*The Social Self*
Vol. 19. R.P. LIBERMAN–*A Guide to Behavioral Analysis & Therapy*
Vol. 22. H.B. PEPINSKY & M.J. PATTON–*The Psychological Experiment: A Practical Accomplishment*
Vol. 23. T.R. YOUNG–*New Sources of Self*
Vol. 24. L.S. WATSON, JR.–*Child Behavior Modification: A Manual for Teachers, Nurses, and Parents*
Vol. 25. H.L. NEWBOLD–*The Psychiatric Programming of People: Neo-Behavioral Orthomolecular Psychiatry*
Vol. 26. E.L. ROSSI–*Dreams and the Growth of Personality: Expanding Awareness in Psychotherapy*
Vol. 27. K.D. O'LEARY & S.G. O'LEARY–*Classroom Management: The Successful Use of Behavior Modification*
Vol. 28. K.A. FELDMAN–*College and Student: Selected Readings in the Social Psychology of Higher Education*
Vol. 29. B.A. ASHEM & E.G. POSER–*Adaptive Learning: Behavior Modification with Children*
Vol. 30. H.D. BURCK *et al.*–*Counseling and Accountability: Methods and Critique*
Vol. 31. N. FREDERIKSEN *et al.*–*Prediction of Organizational Behavior*
Vol. 32. R.B. CATTELL–*A New Morality from Science: Beyondism*
Vol. 33. M.L.WEINER–*Personality: The Human Potential*

TITLES IN THE PERGAMON GENERAL PSYCHOLOGY SERIES (Continued)

Vol. 34. R.M. LIEBERT, J.M. NEALE & E.S. DAVIDSON–*The Early Window: Effects of Television on Children and Youth*
Vol. 35. R. COHEN *et al.*–*Psych City: A Simulated Community*
Vol. 36. A.M. GRAZIANO–*Child Without Tomorrow*
Vol. 37. R.J. MORRIS–*Perspectives in Abnormal Behavior*
Vol. 38. W.R. BALLER–*Bed Wetting: Origins and Treatment*
Vol. 40. T.C. KAHN, J.T. CAMERON, M.B. GIFFEN–*Methods and Evaluation in Clinical and Counseling Psychology*
Vol. 41. M.H. SEGALL–*Political Psychology*
Vol. 42. G.W. FAIRWEATHER *et al.*–*Creating Change in Mental Health Organizations*
Vol. 43. R.C. KATZ & S. ZLUTNICK–*Behavior Therapy and Health Care: Principles and Applications*
Vol. 44. D.A. EVANS & W.L. CLAIBORN–*Mental Health Issues and the Urban Poor*
Vol. 45. K.P. HILLNER–*Learning: A Conceptual Approach*
Vol. 46. T.X. BARBER. N.P. SPANOS & J.F. CHAVES–*Hypnosis, Imagination and Human Potentialities*
Vol. 47. B. POPE–*Interviewing*
Vol. 48 L. PELTON–*The Psychology of Nonviolence*
Vol. 49. K.M. COLBY–*Artificial Paranoia–A Computer Simulation of Paranoid Processes*
Vol. 50. D.M. GELFAND & D.P. HARTMANN–*Child Behavior Analysis and Therapy*
Vol. 51. J.E. TROPMAN *et al.*–*Strategic Perspectives on Social Policy*
Vol. 52. F.H. KANFER & A.P. GOLDSTEIN–*Helping People Change: A Textbook of Methods*
Vol. 53. K. DANZIGER–*Interpersonal Communication*
Vol. 54. P.A. KATZ–*Towards the Elimination of Racism*
Vol. 55. A.P. GOLDSTEIN & N. STEIN–*Prescriptive Psychotherapies*
Vol. 56. M. HERSEN & D.H. BARLOW–*Strategies for Studying Behavior Change*
Vol. 57. J. MONAHAN–*Community Mental Health and the Criminal Justice System*
Vol. 58. R.G. WAHLER, A.E. HOUSE & E.E. STAMBAUGH III–*Ecological Assessment of Child Behavior: A Clinical Package for Home, School, and Institutional Settings*
Vol. 59. P.A. MAGARO–*The Construction of Madness – Emerging Conceptions and Interventions into the Psychotic Process*
Vol. 60. P.M. MILLER–*The Behavioral Treatment of Alcoholism*
Vol. 61. J.P. FOREYT–*Behavioral Treatments of Obesity*